The
F.A.S.T.
Diet (Families Always Succeed Together)

The F.A.S.T. Diet
(Families Always Succeed Together)

The Dean family lost 500 pounds.
Now you can lose weight—and
keep it off—with their simple plan.

TONY DEAN

Harmony Books / New York

Published in the United States by Harmony Books, an imprint of the Crown
Publishing Group, a division of Random House, Inc., New York.
www.crownpublishing.com

Harmony Books is a registered trademark and the Harmony Books colophon is a
trademark of Random House, Inc.

Library of Congress Cataloging-in-Publication Data

Dean, Tony, 1970–
The F.A.S.T. diet (Families Always Succeed Together): the Dean family lost
500 pounds. Now you can lose weight–and keep it off–with their simple plan. /
Tony Dean.–1st ed.
1. Dean, Tony, 1970–Health.   2. Overweight persons–Nebraska–Biography.
3. Overweight persons–Family relationships–Nebraska.   4. Reducing diets.
5. Weight loss.   I. Title.
RC628.D427 2008
362.196'3980092–dc22   2007031712

ISBN 978-0-307-39633-4

Printed in the United States of America

Design by Meryl Sussman Levavi

10 9 8 7 6 5 4 3 2 1

First Edition

Contents

The F.A.S.T. Diet

(Families Always Succeed Together)

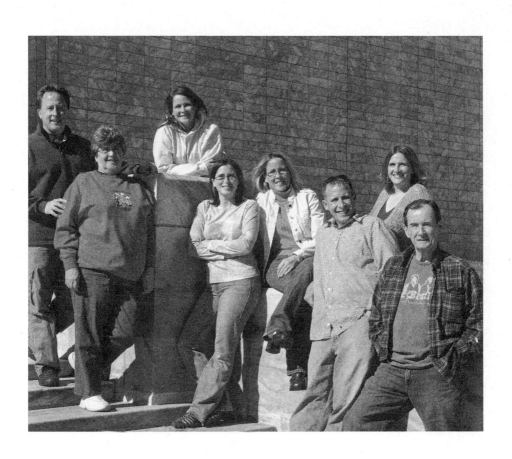

Introduction

In November 2005, an Omaha, Nebraska, family was extremely overweight and unbelievably out of shape. Twelve months later, they had lost more than 500 pounds. They did not take diet pills, eat special foods, count points, or buy any fancy equipment. This family—who managed to overcome a lifetime of weight problems to achieve such remarkable results—is *my* family.

Every day someone asks me, "What is your family's secret? How did you do it?" If I had to sum it up in one word, I'd say *teamwork*! But there's a lot more to it. Let me tell you our amazing story so that you will not only learn how we did it but also be able to do it, too.

At the beginning of those twelve months, we were very short and very round: on average five feet four inches tall and 227.5 pounds. We were hardworking middle-class people just trying to make a living. None of us were ex–college athletes; in fact, none of us had even graduated from college.

The ages, weights, and heights of the eight participants were:

Mike (Dad)	59 years old	271.5 pounds	5′6″
Sheila (Mom)	55 years old	265.0 pounds	5′2″
Tony	35 years old	206.0 pounds	5′7″
Tracy	32 years old	148.0 pounds	5′1″
Tina	31 years old	164.0 pounds	5′2″
Jamie	29 years old	298.0 pounds	5′4″
Jeremy	25 years old	240.5 pounds	5′8″
Julie	24 years old	226.5 pounds	5′0″

We were a family of fatties! Being the royal family of Fatland has always come easy for us. We live in a "small town" of about one million people called Omaha, Nebraska. Our city is one of the nicest places in the world if you like low crime, a moderate cost of living, and high taxes. But for some reason, the people of Omaha are consistently at the top of the charts for being overweight. I suppose we're heavy because it gets so cold and we can't get outside as much as people in other cities do. Sounds like an excuse, doesn't it? It probably is, but it allowed our family to stay fat and unhealthy in the land of so many who were just like us.

Everyone in the Dean family had at one time or another tried to diet—some on our own, others by joining programs—and every one of us had failed. There were a few temporary successes, but in three decades there had never been a single time when I could look at my family as a unit and think, We are healthy. Instead, I thought, I'm scared. How are Mom and Dad going to live in their older years? I knew their lives would be filled with pain and suffering. Given the way they took care of their bodies—or, rather, didn't—there was simply no other possibility.

You are probably reading this book because you want to get healthy. Perhaps you, too, have dieted and failed or worry about your quality of life as you get older. You may have concerns about the health of your spouse, your family, or a friend. Don't worry—this book can transform not only your health but also that of your friends and family. I will share my family's story and show you how we maintained our motivation to eat right and exercise every day. That's right: I said *every day.*

Right now I am sure you are thinking, Every day! Are you kidding me? I'm too busy to exercise every day—I have way too much going on. Did I keep the receipt for this book? Well, don't lose faith yet. Just to prove that almost anyone can lose weight successfully using this program, once we had achieved our goals, we decided to help one hundred random people do the same thing over the course of a year. All of them, like you, "had way too much going on." But now, all of them are succeeding and getting healthy on our program. We can help you overcome the most common obstacles to weight loss. You will quickly realize that many of the problems we share are the same problems you have been battling for years.

I will show you not only how to make the right decisions about food and exercise but also how to stay motivated. There is so much bad information out there about food, and with one "expert" contradicting the next, how do we figure out the truth? I will share our eating plan and tell you what we did that works so that you can do it, too. With balance, you can eat healthy foods that you like, feel full, have more energy, look great, and build confidence in yourself that you never knew you had. And once you have this balance, exercise will be something you cannot live without, instead of something you dread.

But the most important thing you'll learn is how to create a team that will keep you motivated and hold you accountable. On the F.A.S.T. diet, you will learn how to stay healthy once and for all and be a positive role model for those around you. Until you experience it, you can't imagine how good it feels to be a person who motivates someone else to get healthy. Many of the people my family has helped will tell you that their greatest joy is helping others succeed. This is exactly what happened to my family, once the word about what we were doing got out in our community.

Looking back, it seemed as if we blinked and a year had passed. My family of eight had lost 501 pounds, and we decided that we were going to try to share what we had learned with others. We figured that if we could do this, being the kings and queens of Fatland, others could, too. We called a few radio stations and our local news channels, but no one was interested.

Then, almost without warning, there was a media frenzy: every time my phone rang, it was someone new wanting to cover the story. Our local ABC affiliate, Channel 7, was the first to interview my family. None of my family members had ever been on TV before, so they were terribly nervous, but they did great. When our story, "Family Loses 500 Pounds," ran the next night, we loved it. We really thought it sent the message we were trying to convey. Interviews with other local channels followed, and our story soon went national.

Then someone suggested that we call *Good Morning America* to see if they wanted to cover our story. It took a lot of effort, but I finally found *GMA*'s general number and called it.

I had no idea what to do or what to say when someone answered, "ABC News. Can I help you?" I quickly blurted out, "Hi. My name is Tony Dean. I am calling from Omaha, Nebraska, and my family lost five hundred pounds last year, and we want to get this story on *GMA* so we can help people get healthy. Who do I need to talk to?" I caught my breath. There was a short pause before Gloria, the receptionist, said, "You need to talk to me! I need to lose, like, thirty pounds." Then we both laughed.

For the next ten minutes we talked about her situation and her family; she had the same problems we all have: cash crunch, family conflicts, not enough time, and so on. I told her we would help her if she could connect me to someone who knew what to do with this story. "Hold on a second," she said. "I know who you need to talk to."

She put me through to the right person, and soon *Good Morning America* was interested in having us on the show. They flew my whole family to New York in January 2007 to shoot our story in front of a live audience.

Robin Roberts interviewed us; she was a pro and seemed to have a real soft spot for our story. Robin asked a lot of familiar questions: "What is the secret?" "How did you stay motivated?" "How does this team concept work?" She was amazed that a group of people who had failed at dieting their whole lives could suddenly all have success at the same time. The entire segment ran for a little more than six minutes.

When we were finished shooting at *GMA,* we thanked everyone, took a bunch of pictures, and headed out to do some sightseeing: for the next eight hours we went to the Statue of Liberty, Central Park, and Rockefeller Center. At the end of the day, we jumped in the limo, headed to the airport, and started our trip back to Omaha. On the way home, I started to feel as if we had reached the end of this journey, and then I thought, We can't stop here. I believe that in business or fitness or anything else in life, you are either growing or dying; if this was going to be it, then we would surely lose our momentum and, well, who knew what would happen. So I came up with a crazy idea: let's help Omaha get healthy. Let's donate all our free time this year to helping others get fit.

The idea seemed a little wild and maybe even impossible. For the next week or so I let it roll around in my head, then one morning, without telling anyone else in my family, I called Kathy Sarantos-Niver from the local CBS affiliate, Channel 3, and said, "Kathy, we have decided to help one hundred people in this city lose weight.

We are going to do it for free and we need your help rounding up the volunteers." Kathy said, "That sounds great, Tony. I'll be over in thirty minutes."

I decided that the goal would be to get one hundred volunteers to lose 2,500 pounds by the end of 2007. We would have them do everything my family did. We would create teams, whose members would have daily check-ins, write everything down in a diet journal, and exercise each day just like we did. We received twenty or so e-mails from the TV interview with Kathy, and several of those people joined the program. Word spread very quickly after that.

It surprised me how easy it was for people to recruit others. Many people who called said, "I don't think I know anyone who would want to be on my team," but within a day they would ask, "Can my mom join? How about my brother? And I have three coworkers who are interested." One person who said she had no one to ask ended up with twelve people on her team. Soon, even my uncles and aunts became involved. "I think I would like my church to do this," one of my uncles said. He presented the idea at Trinity Church in Omaha, and soon eight men were getting healthy. Within weeks, those eight men became twenty, and a month later the twenty men inspired fifteen women in the church to join. A week later, the local power company called and asked to join. I felt as if I were spreading a virus to people—a good one, the virus of health.

After five weeks, one hundred people had signed up and weighed in at a grand total of 21,812 pounds. The whole process was moving along smoothly. We quickly realized that it was going to be easier to help people lose weight than to administrate the process. By eight weeks into the program, our one hundred people had lost 1,465.7 pounds, and the results were amazing. People contacted me every day to keep me posted on their progress.

"I have been struggling with my weight for years and it just kept creeping up. I have tried lots of things and even though I know they could have worked, I couldn't get motivated until now, with your program. I'm journaling, which I never did with other programs. I'm exercising. I'm thinking about everything that goes in my mouth. I'm reading about nutritional values on everything (driving my husband crazy–not really, he is glad I am doing this).

"I even bought a chocolate muffin the other day, ate a few bites of it and then PITCHED IT in the trash (and I have never done that–chocolate!!!–am I crazy?). And the best part of this is I am having fun and feeling committed to doing this for me and the team. All I know is that I was praying for help and here comes the Dean Family! What a blessing and I thank you all."

—SUZY, OMAHA, NE

"I told your mom yesterday that this program is having a residual effect on my fiancé! I think I told you that he lost over 80 lbs on his own about 6 years ago and has kept it off. He's been content to stay around 210 or less, based on what his cardiologist told him after he lost all the weight. He's been bouncing between 208 and 210 for 6 years. However, the other morning after my weigh-in, he stepped on the scale and was shocked to see he had dropped to 203! He has lost 5 lbs in the past two weeks without thinking about it! We decided that it's because we aren't having extras like guacamole when we go to Mexican restaurants, etc. He's so buzzed! His optimum weight is 189 and now he feels like he can get there just by being supportive of me!

"I so look forward to your e-mails filled with encouragement and tips! Thank you again for allowing me to be a part of your 'family'!"

—CATHY, OMAHA, NE

"You and your family are so AWESOME! I knew when I decided to be on the team that I was destined for greatness, but I never imagined that becoming a new me would feel even the slightest bit like I do right now. I truly credit so much to the accountability factor involved, and the kindness of your family to freely share this with others :) There are still kind and wonderful people in this world that truly are helpful for completely unselfish reasons, and you & your family are just those folks :)

"I know that even though I do have cancer, I am going to beat this again and be the healthiest and strongest I EVER have been! Even way back when, when I was in the Air Force, I only exercised once a year when we did our 'fun-run,' the mile and a half run that was a requirement to pass or be on the 'fat-boy' program. I am exercising daily now and as I mentioned get so FRUSTRATED when I can't make it to the gym . . . LOL Who would have ever guessed it! I am looking forward to progressing through this and becoming the healthiest that I can possibly be :) And even when I reach my goal weight, I know what to do if I do start to gain again. And with healthier eating habits and continued exercise, that should not even be an issue. This is a LIFE CHANGE, not a DIET :) Thank you for your caring and willingness to work along with my doctors through this too; that means so much to me & to my family. The docs are just blown away and really happy with my progress so far and I am MUCH stronger now to fight this. YEAH!"

—MARY, OMAHA, NE

Although the average diet has a success rate of only about 10 percent, the F.A.S.T. diet's is closer to 90 percent. Only a few people have dropped out; everyone else is fighting the battle to get healthy—and winning! The key to success is adding accountability to diet and exercise. You are no different from any of our one hundred participants: you can do it, too.

One of our team players has ten children and still finds time to exercise every day; another is blind. One woman who works three jobs often calls me after her last shift: "Tony, it's three a.m. and I just got done with my workout. Sorry I am checking in so late." People with cancer have joined us, and a few with diabetes don't have it anymore thanks to the F.A.S.T. diet. Nineteen-year-olds who are going to school and trying to start their careers and sixty-five-year-old women on disability all exercise every day and follow the program.

After a few months of success with our group of one hundred volunteers, the American Heart Association called and asked us to get involved with them. They loved our message and thought we could work together to promote good health and exercise in the Omaha area. Soon we were giving speeches and cutting ribbons with the mayor to open walking paths in the city. You may think that the recognition is the best part, but it is nothing compared with being able to help people each day.

As the team lost more and more weight, other family members and friends saw our success and wanted to join, too. My sister Tracy's husband jumped in and quickly went from 188.5 pounds to 156.2. It was so easy for him because Tracy was already doing it. Before long he looked like the lean marine that she had married. The father of my sister Julie's daughter has type II diabetes. Before beginning the F.A.S.T. program, he was on several medications and had to check his blood sugar frequently. His diet was terrible, and his blood sugar was always above 300. After spending three weeks on the program and consulting with his doctor, he saw his blood sugar drop to the 90s. He couldn't believe it. My amazing mother-in-law, Kathy, got involved several months after we started the F.A.S.T. diet and has lost 23.6 pounds so far: her goal weight is only ten pounds away. She has not been this thin in more than twenty years.

As more people joined, we realized something fantastic: the F.A.S.T. diet worked! By teaching people to work together we were able to transform a lifetime of dieting failure into instant success. We found out how to turn people who *can't* do it alone into people who *can* do it together.

Exciting things continue to happen, and I now realize that this good fortune is a product of the real "Golden Rule" of life. No, not "He who has the gold makes the rules." The one I am talking about is "Everyone wants to get something in life—good health, money, fame—but to get anything you must give first. It is this act of giving that allows you to finally get what you really want." Maybe it is time for you to start giving: give good health to yourself and give the knowledge you will get from reading this book to those around you. Give your friends, your family, and your coworkers an opportunity to get healthy by watching you start to succeed on your path to fitness.

You can do it, too.

Chapter 1

THE F.A.S.T. DIET:
HOW IT ALL STARTED

About three months before we started the F.A.S.T. diet, I was
working in my home office in the Millard subdivision of
Omaha. (F.A.S.T. stands for Families Always Succeed Together. It
has nothing to do with speed–though if you stick to it you will see
results quickly!–or with fasting, as in not eating.) Julie, my youngest
sister, worked as my assistant, and we had a little office set up in my
basement. When we weren't working, we loved to watch the hit TV
show *The Biggest Loser.* I was amazed to see how fast other fatties
like us were losing weight. (You should know that in the F.A.S.T.
diet lexicon, "fatty" is an endearing term, not an offensive one. The
message behind the word *fatty* is "We love you, now do something
about being fat!")

However, as we watched these TV fatties get thinner and thinner, I couldn't help but notice that the participants were in an ideal
environment for losing weight. They got permission to leave their
jobs and families for three months and do nothing but work out

with the best trainers money could buy at a world-class facility on a beautiful mountain with hills to climb and a forest to hike. When the contestants returned home, gym equipment and a new fridge filled with all the right foods were waiting. If that wasn't enough, they were competing for a $250,000 prize, and the entire world was watching them—talk about accountability! I remember one episode in which a contestant sneaked down to the kitchen at 2:00 a.m. and took a brownie out of the fridge. As she carefully looked around to make sure no one was watching, the music from *Jaws* kicked in. You could just feel the entire world gasp–"Whoa!"–when she took a bite.

With all of this support and accountability, not to mention the possibility of a great reward, how could the contestants not lose weight on that show? The only better motivation I can think of would be a treadmill that worked like an ATM—each time you burned a calorie it would spit out a $20 bill. Wouldn't you love a machine like that? And wouldn't you love to have all the help and privileges enjoyed by TV show contestants?

Unfortunately, losing weight in real life is exactly the opposite. Average, hardworking people struggle to afford a gym membership, never mind top-dollar trainers who charge between $50 and $250 for a training session. Most of us would lose our jobs if we took three months off to lose weight. As for food, where do I start? On nearly every corner is a fast-food place more than happy to sell you a burger and a shake that total 300 calories more than what you need to consume for the entire day. In the real world, temptations are everywhere.

However much we envy the contestants on *The Biggest Loser,* they still have a powerful lesson to teach us: even though they have been given every advantage and put into the perfect setting to lose weight, they still cry and complain, "I can't do it." When I first heard them say this, I wanted to scream at the TV, "What do you mean, you can't do it? What other advantages do you want?" But then one day, while my sister and I were discussing the show, I realized an important truth about losing weight—it isn't easy, even in an ideal situation. This realization led me to the secret to losing weight: accountability. Since losing weight is so difficult, you just can't do it alone. You need to be part of a team that will help you follow through when you are weak and not able to do it by yourself.

The contestants on *The Biggest Loser* had a lot of people watching them, and this motivated them to keep going. And then I had a brainstorm—I couldn't get a TV audience to watch me and keep me motivated and accountable, but I could get my family to do it. In fact, we could all do it for each other. I could create a program for my family so that none of us would ever have to struggle with our weight again.

I turned to my sister and said, "Hey, Julie, I have an idea. What if we were to create our own weight-loss program? We could call it 'The Dean Family's F.A.S.T. Diet,' for Families Always Succeed Together. I could learn everything we need to know about food and exercise, and then we could get the whole family together and present it to them.

"The secret to this show has nothing to do with weight loss and has everything to do with support and accountability," I went on. "So we need to create teams that each person must check in with every day. If anyone starts to slip, they have to call their teammate and say, 'Help! I'm just about to eat a whole pizza by myself!' It would be the teammate's job to help them through their weak moment."

Thinking some more, I said, "We could take pictures every week and weigh in every Saturday, and I could create a simple website with before and after pictures." I paused for a minute to wait for Julie's response to my idea. She was floored!

"If you don't do it, I will!" she said. She was glowing and could barely work for the rest of the day. That didn't work out so well for me, because, as I said, she was my assistant. But despite all our excitement and enthusiasm, we did the worst thing we could have done. We procrastinated and did nothing.

Three or four months passed, and every once in a while one of us would bring up my idea again, but still we did nothing. (People are capable of doing great things, but sometimes, even when that greatness is right in front of us, we persist in doing nothing.) Finally, one night in November 2005, the whole family was at a birthday party at my parents' home. Julie came to me and said, "Maybe we should present your idea to the group." I was tempted to procrastinate some more, but I thought about the huge potential health benefits for the people I love the most and that got me motivated. I asked my parents and siblings to meet me in a back room for five minutes. We handed the kids to our spouses and went to my parents' room. I can still remember the moment as if it were yesterday: a group of overweight and unhealthy people looked back at me, everyone in loose pants or sweats and shirts so tight the buttons were about to pop off. We looked pitiful.

I made my announcement: "I have figured out the missing ingredient to successful dieting, and I now know why diets fail. I have also figured out a way that we can all be as fit and healthy as we have ever been in twelve months, and then maybe we can motivate the world to do the same thing. We could spend the rest of our lives being thin and healthy, all the while helping millions of other people to achieve the same goals. We could become role models for our kids and relatives and inspire them to live healthy lives. We could all become the people we really want to be."

Almost everyone was looking at me wide-eyed. There were two skeptics, my dad and my sister Tracy. But everyone else was ready to hear more right away.

"There are several problems with dieting today," I went on. "First, there is so much information, much of it incorrect, and there is almost no way to tell what is true and what is not. I can tell everyone exactly what they should and shouldn't eat." (This wasn't exactly true. I wasn't crystal-clear about nutrition at that point, but I knew I could quickly learn what I needed to know.) "I also know what each of us needs to do for exercise, depending on our age and current fitness level." (I had spent over $12,000 on more than two hundred personal training sessions, so I was pretty familiar with what kind of exercises we would need to do.) "Last, I will show everyone how many calories they need to eat in a day to lose weight and remain healthy. Then, we will all write down what we eat each day and track exactly what is going into our bodies.

"The final piece is actually the family itself or, better yet, the team that our family will become. We are very fortunate to have an amazingly close family. We need to use our greatest resource, which is each other. We will create one big team of eight, then each week we will break the team into two-person teams. Every other week we will rotate partners for variety. If anyone is tempted to cheat on their diet or exercise, they always have to call a teammate first and ask permission. Your teammate is responsible for trying to talk you out of cheating, but if he or she can't, then you can cheat. Every day you will have to schedule a time to call your teammate and talk about what you did the day before and go over your numbers. Finally, we will weigh in every Saturday at 8:00 a.m. and track our results. What do you think?"

The reaction was pure excitement. Even the skeptics were excited (although still a bit skeptical).

"Let's talk about it over the next couple of days and decide when we are going to start. After all, the holidays are coming up, and we can't be dieting around the holidays. We are fatties, loyal to our fatty traditions." Of course, putting off the choice of when to start was more procrastination. The idea could have died right there, but fortunately the fire never cooled. The whole family was talking nonstop about my idea.

Finally, almost everyone agreed to start at the first of the year. Looking back, I think, Are you kidding me? If that had been our final decision, we never would have made it. I've learned since then that when to start a new program is always an issue once you have decided to lose weight. After all, you can't start in November, because there is Thanksgiving, right? December isn't good, because there are more holidays. January naturally seems like the best time since it is the start of a new year, but it never works out because suddenly you get very busy at your job again after all the days off. It's too hard to get to the gym in February because of the snow. One excuse follows another, and pretty soon it's November again.

A few days after our first meeting, I called everyone in the group and said, "If we are going to do this, we've got to do it now." They all agreed. On November 30, we would meet at my house for a weigh-in, a videotaping, and pictures. If we were ever going to learn to control ourselves, having a thirty-day head start before Christmas made a lot of sense to me. It was a beautiful sight when everyone showed up on that day, like looking at a blank canvas and being the only one who really knew that it was about to become a Monet.

Each time someone stepped on the scale, you could see how disappointed he or she was. But it didn't matter; we were all there for each other. The teamwork started right away: "That's all right, Jamie. You can do it." But we still wondered how we had let ourselves get this heavy. Why had we settled for these overweight, out-of-shape bodies?

I was the cameraman and the interviewer for the individual pictures and videos. I had created a set of questions to ask my family, and their responses were unbelievably similar. Each of us had unique issues, but we shared many of the same problems. Most of us had sore backs and knees, and we all got winded when we went up a flight of stairs. We were all afraid that we were being terrible role models for our kids.

When I finished videotaping, I was amazed at how we all shared the same goals. We wanted to lose weight. We wanted to get healthy. We wanted to be good role models. We didn't want to live at the doctor's office when we were sixty years old. As individuals, we had never made any real progress toward these goals. But now that we were a team, things were about to change drastically.

Chapter 2

MEET THE TEAM: OUR STORY

Something amazing happens when a team of like-minded individuals works together toward the same goal. People always talk about the synergy that is created when a team gets together, but in all my years in the business world I had never really seen it in action until my family started getting fit.

The fantastic people who I am lucky enough to call my family are not really special in any way—they are typical working-class Americans. When you read their stories, you will probably relate to one or more of them on a very personal level, or at least relate to the problems that we all share.

Losing weight is a *battle:* you have to fight if you are going to win. It is not easy. You cannot treat it as a casual endeavor; there is no quick fix, but if you approach weight loss with the right attitude and the right team, it is a battle that you must and can win.

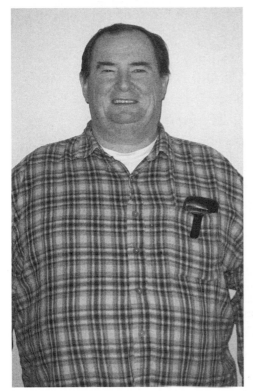 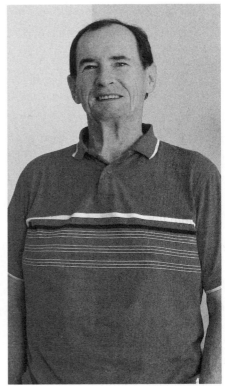

Mike Dean

Age at start of program: 59

Height: 5'6"

Starting weight: 271.5 pounds

Current weight: 170.0 pounds (goal weight)

My dad was fifty-nine years old when we started the F.A.S.T. diet. He is now sixty and has lost 101.5 pounds. When I was growing up, Mike was the best example of what *not to do* if you wanted to be healthy. He was always a loving, caring father and a role model in more ways than one, but never when it came to food or exercise. He made it to every Pee Wee soccer game even though he worked seventy hours a week; however, when it came to participating in sports himself, he just could not do it.

I remember one time several years ago when he tried to shoot baskets with me, and a game of H-O-R-S-E quickly turned into one-on-one. I was so excited because my dad never did that kind of thing. He was so overweight that I just assumed he couldn't play on the basketball court with me. But before I knew it, he was running and dribbling and playing basketball. I was smiling ear to ear.

Unfortunately, my happiness was interrupted about forty-five seconds into the game. Suddenly my dad started wheezing and coughing. He bent over like he was going to pass out or have a heart attack. His physical condition was so bad that he couldn't run around a 10×10-foot cement square with a two-pound basketball for a full minute. It made me very sad. I said, "Thanks for trying," and he went inside to rest. That was twenty-three years ago—he was only thirty-seven.

In many ways, my dad was the typical American male. He went to work, came home and spent some time with his kids, had dinner, and then wound down from the day with a six-pack or two while watching hours and hours of TV. He would almost always stay up late, relaxing in his easy chair until 2:00 or 3:00 a.m. while snacking on Nestlé Crunch bars, Reese's peanut butter cups, and other super-high-calorie foods. It was always a standing joke that our father had no neck. Looking back, it really wasn't that funny because he didn't.

Now, he is in the greatest shape of his life. When he goes to the gym, no one works out harder than he does. My family's program has completely transformed him. My dad will get on the floor and roll around with my three-year-old son. Nothing seems to tire either of them out. Mike has always been a happy guy who is easy to get along with, but now he's a role model for fitness. Everyone he works with is blown away by his results. None of his old friends recognize him. One day, my dad showed my three-year-old niece Emilie a picture of himself taken the year before, when he was still a fatty.

"Emilie, who is that?" Dad asked.

"Papa, that was you when you were old," Emilie said.

I laugh every time I hear that story. Consider how getting healthy could impact you and the memories you create with your kids or nieces and nephews or grandchildren. What kind of a role model are you now? Think about how much better you'll be when you transform your health and your body through the F.A.S.T. program. You can even positively affect people you have never met! Everyone wants to be healthy, and, as my dad's story illustrates, it's never too late!

Mike Dean

When I started the F.A.S.T. diet, my body didn't have the slightest clue what a workout was. I hadn't exercised for over thirty years. My heart, lungs, and muscles all had to go back to work. No more lounging around.

The first month I slowly worked myself into it by doing mainly cardio, and I saw small improvements. After just a short period of time my results started adding up, and I became highly motivated and driven to beat my own records on different machines. It didn't matter to me that my records were low; they were *my* records. During the first couple of weeks, I was burning maybe 200 calories in a workout, which was great for a fifty-nine-year-old man after thirty years of doing nothing. Now, I am burning between 800 and 900 calories in an hour on almost all the machines I work out on. I am also lifting three times the weight I started out with.

I go to the gym every day religiously because I enjoy it. Don't get me wrong, it is not easy, but it is very fulfilling to me. It's kind of like a carpenter building a house: as he goes along he steps back and looks at his work and is very pleased with himself. This is my exact feeling. I look better; I feel better; I'm stronger; I'm more coordinated; I'm more flexible; I can breathe easier—this is the house that I'm working on.

My personal goal for a one-hour workout now is to burn 700 to 750 calories per day regardless of what machine I use. I usually beat that number and I am never under. Even if I have to work an extra ten minutes to get there, I do it because I remember when I used to feel unhealthy and I would much rather feel the way I do now. The exercise is no longer a burden because it makes me feel good.

As the weeks pass, the minimum number of calories I will accept for a workout grows. I also try to work a different machine every day, because I think it is important to get outside of your comfort zone. Some of my best workouts were on machines I had learned to use that day. One day a week I pick a machine and go on a mission to break one of my personal records.

Another way to stay motivated is to keep trying to master different machines. The first time I worked out on the cross-trainer I thought, This is impossible. After thirty seconds on it I felt like my legs were ready to collapse. A week later I was was up to two and a half minutes, then ten to fifteen minutes; after a month I could work out for one hour on level 10, and I am still getting better. The secret is not to have a big workout today or work yourself so hard that you can't walk for the next three days. The secret is simply to track what you did today and try to do a little better tomorrow.

Each time I get on a new machine, after that first thirty seconds, my mind will start saying, Maybe you should try a different machine; this is too hard. During my first few months of exercise, I would remind myself that the month before I couldn't even walk on a treadmill; this encouragement would help me get over my doubts and have a great workout. Getting healthy is about tiny improvements each day. Small steps will yield faster results than you realize.

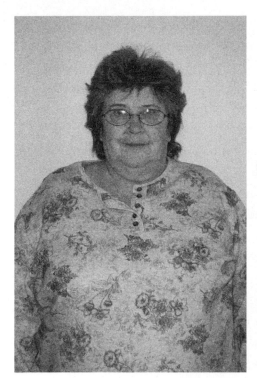 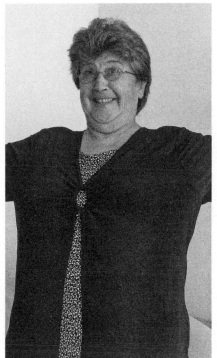

I really don't expect to be able to keep up with my kids using these machines and weights, but my personal goals and successes are plenty for me. I can't believe I waited this long to get serious about my health, but I will tell you this—I will never go back. Life is not only short, but it is great when you give yourself a chance to enjoy it.

Sheila Dean
Age at start of program: 55
Height: 5′2″
Starting weight: 265.0 pounds
Current weight: 200.6 pounds (goal weight: 148.0 pounds)

The first night we discussed this diet and our plan to get healthy, my mom was on cloud nine. The family literally had to hold her down to keep her from running right to the gym at 10 p.m. or whatever time it was when we talked. This enthusiasm is typical of my mom (and me, too).

In the past, she would get all excited about something new and be totally into it. Then as the novelty of the idea wore off, so did her passion for it. In this world of constant "new this" and "new that" it can be hard to maintain your focus. If this sounds like you, then you can learn a lot from my mother.

When we started the program, she was fifty-five years old, and her profession had not changed for the last thirty-five years: she took care of all the kids. In fact, she still does, except now she has nine grandkids whom she watches all day long. We have tried many times to commit her to an institution for agreeing to watch nine kids for ten hours a day, but the authorities seem to think it is legal. I have always wondered how anyone could maintain her sanity in this environment. But she does.

Mom's weight problem started, as it does for many women, after her first pregnancy. As a schoolgirl, she was always thin. Then she graduated, got married, and had six children over the next ten years. This gave her almost no time between babies to lose the weight. It wasn't long before her weight was out of control and she became a fatty.

Mom had tried at least a dozen diets with only limited success. Each time she would lose some weight. Soon after, she would lose all interest in dieting and the weight would come right back.

Obviously, I have never been a woman, but I counsel women in the F.A.S.T. program, and it seems to me that the problem is not just the weight a woman gains during pregnancy but also the hectic schedules (hers and her child's) that leave her less time to exercise and eat right.

Midway through the F.A.S.T. diet, my mom had several weeks when her weight stayed exactly the same or within a few pounds. She really struggled to maintain her momentum. I know there are many people who have the same problem. The lesson Sheila Dean gives us is this: *Have fewer kids.*

Of course, I am joking. The real lesson is, We all need help. Once you understand this, you can find a team or someone to help you who wants what you want. You get help by asking for help, which in turn helps not only you and your teammate but also everyone who is watching you succeed.

My mom quickly learned how to make the support of the team work for her. Without realizing it, she became the person who proves that *it can be done.* If you stop trying to be an island and ask for a little help, you can succeed and be a role model.

I had never seen my mother exercise before she joined the F.A.S.T. diet. Never! I had never even seen her going for an exercise-related walk. Now she works out every day at the gym and swims laps. She is a role model for her family and for any woman who says, "I can't do that." Believe me, *you can*!

Sheila Dean

When I was growing up, I always felt like I was a fat person. In October 1968, at the age of seventeen, I got married—I weighed 128 pounds. During that first year of our life together, I had two miscarriages. Then, in 1970, our first child was born, a son, Tony. From 1970 to 1981, I had six kids and one miscarriage. As you can see, for ten years I was always pregnant. The pounds kept adding up, and it seemed that whenever I tried to lose weight I would get pregnant again.

After having all the kids, my body was not exactly a fine-tuned machine anymore. Everyone told me to watch my weight or I would regret it. I wish I had listened to them.

I was always pretty active; with six kids how could I not be? I was an avid bowler and so was my husband. I coached a team for ten years while my girls were in high school. After they all graduated, I gave it up and quit bowling altogether because it bothered my ankles. I couldn't bowl three games at one time anymore; I was too *fat.* My feet couldn't handle my weight. I had to quit something I loved because my body would not allow me to do it anymore.

In 2005 my son Tony came up with an idea to help us all lose weight together. It seemed to him that we had been doing it all wrong. I listened carefully because I was tired of being so overweight for so long. When he said we would be doing it together, I just about jumped up and hugged him. I am not a weak-minded person by any means; in fact, I think most people would say I am too strong. But for some reason losing weight is just one of those things that I could never accomplish. But I knew if I had a team, I could do it.

Losing the 60 pounds I have lost so far has breathed new life into every day. I can do so much more now. I can even run. I will not lie to anyone, though; it is not easy. In fact, it is hard some days to get to the gym when you are tired and just want to sit around and relax. The sacrifice is worth the reward. You simply cannot put a price on your health.

My renewed health has allowed me to take up bowling again. At the start of the bowling season, my grandson joined a league; I took him bowling and bowled for the first time in about twelve years. It felt like I was alive again, not because I could throw a ball down a lane, but because I had the choice to do what I wanted again and I was not restrained by my poor health.

I am so thankful to be a part of this family and encourage anyone who needs to start their journey to health to unite with those around you—family, friends, coworkers, or whoever. You will never regret it.

My weight loss has made me a better grandmother to my nine grandchildren. There are so many more things that I can do now that I couldn't before. It makes my day so much easier now that I'm not so tired all the time and can keep up with all of them. I love to take them all for walks or go to the park. Most of my friends and family say, "I

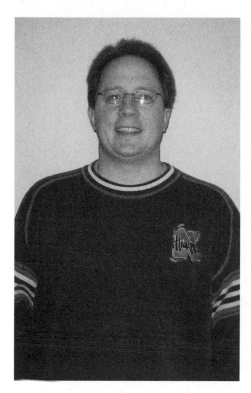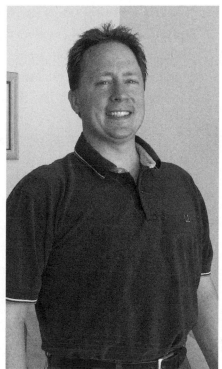

don't know how you do it every day," but I don't know what I would do if I didn't have them. These kids are the love of my life and I want to be around to see them grow up. So this diet that my son has come up with and the accountability it creates have basically saved my life. Plus, it has allowed me to turn the time I already spend with my grandkids into quality time. I wish you luck as you create your team. Achieving your health goals is worth the effort—take my word for it.

Tony Dean
Age at start of program: 35
Height: 5'7"
Starting weight: 206.0
Current weight: 169.8 (goal weight)

I am thirty-five years old now and have always been 20 to 40 pounds overweight. I was never obese, but I was always just fat enough to feel uncomfortable in my clothes and to dread going anywhere that required a bathing suit. I tried many times to get to a reasonable weight, but like my mom I would soon lose interest in dieting.

About halfway through 2006 I hit my goal weight (I now weigh 169.8 pounds). I don't recall ever weighing this little, not even when I met my wife, almost fifteen years ago. Seven years later we married, and I weighed 210 pounds. Isn't it interesting how we almost always gain weight once we get comfortable with a spouse or a significant other? I have found that many people trying to get healthy simply want to weigh what they did on their wedding day. What a great gift to give your spouse: give them back the person they married!

When I started the F.A.S.T. diet, I was probably the fittest member of my family. I could run farther and exercise longer than anyone else in our group. However, I also had a problem: I was in a cast with a torn Achilles tendon. This is a serious injury that can take a year or more to heal completely. When we started the program, I could not walk at all and was having problems with swelling in my leg.

Here I was, telling my family what a great idea it was for them to go to the gym every day, and all I could do was sit on a couch with my leg in the air. I was pushing them to not make excuses and to find solutions. "Find a way to do it!" I told them. But I could not walk except on crutches for a very short distance before I would have to stop and elevate my leg.

So I did exactly what I had been telling them to do: I found a solution. I asked my doctor, "When this cast comes off, can I walk?" He said, "No; you will have to wear a boot for six weeks, and you need to stay off the leg as much as you can." Okay, I thought, this is a serious problem.

"Can I swim?" I asked.

"No," he said. "There is no way you can get in and out of the pool without getting hurt."

"Doc, I have to exercise," I insisted. "What if I promise not to use my legs in the pool? I will drag them through the water when I swim and not kick. I will be careful maneuvering with my crutches in and out of the pool." Finally, he agreed.

For the next couple of months, swimming was all I did. My hair was like straw and I smelled of chlorine twenty-four hours a day, but I kept swimming.

My doctor had said all along that when the cast came off, I was going to have to endure a painful rehab. One day, he pulled me aside and said, "If you want to skip rehab, you can. A guy like you doesn't need it. Your exercise regimen is the best rehab you could have possibly done. Stick with it!" (By the way, I'm 100 percent healed now.)

The lesson is this: At some point, we all have to learn that exercise is important. We can either learn that lesson now, when we can do something about our futures, or we can learn when it is too late; when we are old and feeble and all of our joints have locked up from lack of use. Simply put, we benefit for the rest of our lives from exercising now, or we pay for not doing it later. If *you* don't make the right choice now, advertisers, diet pill companies, and people more interested in your money than in your health will make the wrong one for you.

Once you decide to exercise every day, you need to commit to it. No matter what, you cannot renege. This commitment needs to become a part of you. Life will throw obstacles at you constantly. You will have every reason not to exercise, but you still have to do it.

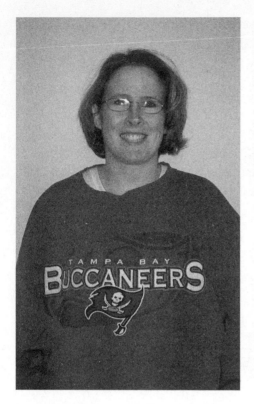 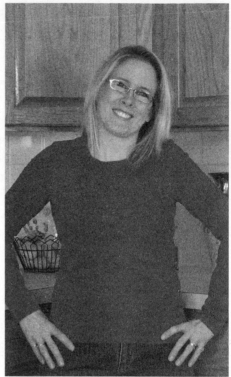

When exercise comes first and you learn to work your life around your health, a big change will take place that you will never regret. The grass will look greener, your food will taste better, and you will be happier and more confident. The world really does seem to be a better place when you take a little time each day for yourself. Devote that time to yourself every day, and you will see changes that you never thought were possible.

Tracy Wright
Age at start of program: 32
Height: 5′1″
Starting weight: 148.0 pounds
Current weight: 115.4 (goal weight)

Do you feel like there is simply not enough time in the day to exercise? Then pay close attention to the story of my oldest sister, Tracy. She somehow manages to juggle more in a day than seems humanly possible. I realize that most people already have an over-booked schedule. But even Tracy found a way to overcome the excuse of "no time for exercise."

Back in 2005 Tracy's day started early in the morning. She was the manager of a children's respite center, a very demanding job that required a fifty-hour-a-week commitment. She was often on call and had to run back and forth to the center at unexpected moments. And she was taking courses and working toward her college degree.

Then there were her three active kids: Kyle (a bowler and a cellist), Ashley (a competitive gymnast), and Ryan (a gymnast). Add in two or three hours of homework every night, and there simply was no time for anything else. Tracy's husband, Jeremey, went to school full-time while working fifty hours a week as an engineer and twelve hours at a second job. When my family started the program, Tracy couldn't imagine doing anything other than what she was already doing. There was certainly no time for her to get to the gym, even if she could have afforded to join, which she couldn't.

Instead of saying it could not be done, Tracy started asking my favorite question, "How can it be done?" She bought a used treadmill for $100 that didn't work very well–but it did work. Early in the morning she would get up and work out before the day started, or she would work out late at night, when everyone else was in bed. No one really wants to get up early or stay up late to work out, but you have to do it if that is your only choice.

Jeremey had a few pounds to lose himself, so he got involved almost immediately. Since they didn't have the money to join a gym, they improvised. Tracy would run up and down the stairs in their basement for thirty to sixty minutes while Jeremey walked or ran on the treadmill. The next night they would switch. Sometimes they would mix in jumping rope or they would alternate activities like running stairs in the middle of the workout.

They did what almost all of us never do—they refused to quit. They knew they had a big problem and had to figure out how to solve it: they did not want to let down the team. They didn't want to be the only ones in the family who didn't follow through and work out. As Tracy's story shows, a good plan for accountability can help you achieve things you never dreamed were possible. You can beat the demons that are stopping you from succeeding.

When Tracy used to run up to the front door of the school to pick up her kids, she would be tired and breathing heavily. A couple of months after she started working out, she was able to sprint up to the school door without breathing hard at all. Once when I was doing a personal training session with her, I asked her to run on the treadmill for ten minutes. I thought she was going to die. But she did it. Four weeks later, she called me and said, "Tony, I just ran for an hour on the treadmill." I could not have been more impressed.

Tracy and Jeremey both lost their excess weight very quickly, and Tracy was the first to reach her goal weight. When she started the diet, she was a size 12. She had been a size 8 in high school but was convinced that her body could never get back to that size again. She now wears a size 4 or 6. When Tracy reached her goal weight, we were all there at our usual Saturday weigh-in. When she stood on the scale, screams and cheers erupted, because we realized that the whole family, not only Tracy, had done something really big. She was the trailblazer who showed everyone else that it could be done.

Tracy was supposed to increase her calories and reduce her exercise a little because now she just wanted to maintain her weight. But at the next weigh-in, the most shocking thing happened when Tracy stepped on the scale—she'd lost another two pounds. I said, "Tracy, you have been working so hard to lose weight that now you can't stop." We laughed, but it was true. She was losing weight by accident. When I tell this story, people always say, "That would be a nice problem to have," and I agree, but the only way you will ever get there is by working hard and being consistent like Tracy.

Tracy increased her calories again and cut back her exercise schedule to three or four days a week; her weight quickly stabilized. She is a great example for people who think they don't have the time to work out or who have to overcome obstacles to exercise. We all think we are busier than the next guy, but we really aren't. When you *really* want to exercise, you will find a way to do it, regardless of your personal obstacles.

Tracy Wright

"Does my butt look fat?" was something I would ask my mom, sisters, friends, whoever was around when I was growing up. The person I asked would always get angry and say something sarcastic like, "Oh yeah, you are *such* a cow." Looking back, I realize that it didn't matter what anyone said: I didn't believe compliments, and I was offended by criticism. Either way, in my mind, I was a cow, and I didn't understand why the people around me were not supportive. I always felt insecure and unsure of my looks and especially my weight. I was the girl who thought she was huge, but the funny thing is, I wore a size 7. It is crazy how your mind can distort your self-image so much that you really have no idea what you look like. I spent most of my teenage years with this distorted image in my head, and it contributed to many other insecurities. I questioned my abilities at school and at work. I couldn't believe that my husband would choose me, a size 7 cow, over so many other beautiful, skinny girls. I was sad and cried often; I was very down on myself. So, when did I finally realize that I hadn't been fat and that I did not have a fat butt after all? When I got *really fat*!

When I was twenty-three, I had my first child. I gained 60 pounds and loved every minute of my pregnancy, until the weight stuck with me. When I delivered my first son, I weighed in at 175 pounds. That is way too much weight for someone my height. I did manage to drop a lot of this weight before baby number 2, but when I was twenty-five, I delivered my daughter after gaining another 60 pounds. This time I weighed in at 184 pounds on the day of delivery. This time the weight stuck, and the answer to the question "Does my butt look fat?" was a definite yes. Actually, while I was pregnant, my mother, whom I love dearly, thought it necessary to inform me that I had a "Big Bertha Butt."

After about a year of very little weight loss and even a little weight gain, I joined a local weight-loss program. It worked, but not in a good way. I did lose weight, but I was always hungry, did not exercise, and learned nothing about what my body needed and how to maintain my weight loss. The loss was short-lived because, wouldn't you know it, I got pregnant again. With baby number 3 I gained 47 pounds because on the advice of my doctor I saw a nutritionist to slow my weight gain. Weighing in at 174 pounds, I delivered my son. I then lost about 20 pounds, and for the next six years my weight has fluctuated between 145 and 155.

Over the past six years I have dieted several times, once getting down to 130 pounds, but very quickly jumping right back up to the 150s. I lacked energy to do things with my kids, at work, and in general. I was eating poorly and not exercising. Even though I was bigger than I really wanted to be, I thought I looked good considering I had given birth to three kids. I thought it did not really matter anyway, since my hips would never go back to the way they were before I had children. I learned to settle for who I was rather than who I wanted to be, or who I could be, and, boy, was I wrong. Those baby hips and chunky thighs *will* fade away. I am a thirty-three-year-old woman with three kids who went from a size 12 to a size 6. My thighs no longer touch when I walk, and *no, my butt is not fat.*

Some of the most important things I learned along the way, and the advice I would give to anyone who is looking to make this change in their life, is to believe in yourself, to use the team to help guide you to reach your goals, and to never settle. If you cheat on your foods or exercise, there is no excuse, and you are letting down yourself and your team. If you choose to work hard and meet all your exercise, food, and teamwork goals, you will find success. I won't lie; this seems simple enough, but it is hard work. You will sweat, cry, and try to trick yourself into quitting, but in the end, you will be healthier and happier and look better than you have ever looked in your life. It is the most worthwhile thing I have ever done, next to having my children (minus the combined 167 pounds that I gained during the three pregnancies). Work hard, never give up, and make it happen.

Tina Chereck

Age at start of program: 31
Height: 5′2″
Starting weight: 164.0
Current weight: 123.2 (goal weight)

Where do I start with my sister Tina? She is strong and sometimes stubborn, always thoughtful but sometimes rash. She is a manager for a chain of BP gas stations in Omaha and is a tremendous success. She is reliable, consistent, and hardworking. When we were younger and I said, "Hey, who wants to jump out of a plane with me?" Tina was the first one in the car.

Unlike most of us, Tina has been very thin most of her life (and we hated her for it . . . just kidding, Tina). As a kid, she was as skinny

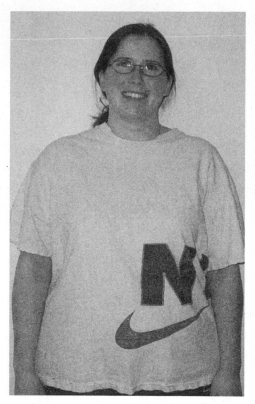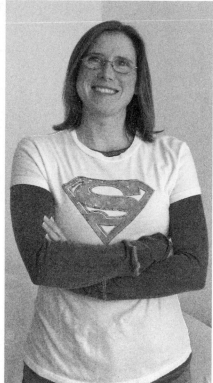

as a rail. I think she weighed less than 105 pounds in high school. Although she was an excellent bowler, she was never into physically demanding sports. Exercise just wasn't her thing, and she didn't need to do it.

After graduating from high school, Tina went to work; she eventually married and had a son, Tyler. Sounds normal, right? Believe me, it wasn't. When Tina got pregnant for the first time, everything was great. Then suddenly all of the joy and excitement unraveled when it turned out she had a medical condition that mimics pregnancy. Tina was devastated.

In many families, having children is a big deal. In my family, if you don't have six kids by the time you are twenty-one, people ask you, "Hey, when are you going to have some kids?" So you can imagine how disappointed Tina was. She jumped on the depression/weight gain roller coaster. And, unfortunately, this roller coaster only went up; she put on several pounds.

Tina struggled for a long time to get over the disappointment; then a miracle happened: she became pregnant for real. Everything went great for five weeks, until the doctors discovered that Tina had a tubal pregnancy. The baby was growing in one of her fallopian tubes instead of in the uterus, and if the pregnancy wasn't terminated, the tube would explode and Tina and her baby would both die.

The choice was to either terminate or lose both her and her baby. This was much worse than what had happened before. Tina fell deeper into depression, and the pounds kept piling on.

However, unlike most sad stories, this one had a happy ending. Her next pregnancy was successful. Tina gave birth to Tyler, a happy, healthy boy. After a miscarriage, Tara, Tina's daughter, was born. Tina never got over the trauma of her losses, though. Even after she had her two wonderful children, she was still depressed; in fact, she took medication for it. And now her petite frame was carrying almost 170 pounds.

In the videotape of our first weigh-in, Tina can't stop crying. She was still suffering emotionally, even though she finally had everything that she wanted. Fortunately, the F.A.S.T. diet was just about to save her life, her sanity, and maybe even her husband's sanity.

Tina slowly started to exercise, and before I knew it, she was jogging. Ten months later, she had achieved her goal weight of 123 pounds. This was not the same Tina, though: she had become a serious runner. In fact, it is not unusual for Tina to run to our weekly weigh-ins on Saturday morning. The distance from her house to mine is seven miles, and more than once she has done it in the pouring rain. She also has finished her first half marathon and ran the thirteen miles in just over two hours.

Within a month of Tina's starting the program, people were asking her, "What are you so excited about?" Her answer was always the same: "I am getting healthy again." Being active helped her get over her depression. Once Tina took back her life, she was still sad about her losses, but now she could handle that sadness. She was taking control of both her health and her life. She was doing something just for her, and it is hard to be depressed when you are healthy and people are telling you that you look great.

Tina's story shows us that tragedy can happen at any time to anyone. You may have been prom queen or prom king before life threw you a curveball. It doesn't matter; the way you climb out of your hole is one step at a time, one day at a time. It won't happen overnight, but if you eat well, stay active, and take care of yourself, it *will* happen. Wallowing in your misery and eating unhealthy foods to comfort yourself will only make things worse. As a friend once told me, "The first thing you do when you find yourself in a hole is to stop digging."

Tina Chereck

I was the one who never had a weight problem growing up. If anything, I would say I was borderline anorexic. I would not allow myself to weigh more than 110 pounds. And even at 110, I still felt like I was heavy! If I did go over 110, I would practically starve myself to get back under that magic number; so I guess I did have a problem, just not the same problem as everyone else.

At twenty-four I found myself unexpectedly pregnant. The pregnancy started out normal: I felt great and had no morning sickness. What I found out quickly, though, was that I could pack on the pounds fairly easily. At sixteen weeks, having gained 20 pounds, I found out that I had a blighted ovum, which causes your body to think and act like it is pregnant, but no fetus actually forms. My boyfriend and I were crushed; we were really just getting used to the idea that we were going to have a baby, and then the doctors told us that it was not going to happen. I had to have a D & C and mourn the loss of a baby that had never actually existed. This was the beginning of my postpartum depression. I recovered from the surgery but never recovered my weight: I was now up to about 130 pounds. That is still not bad for someone who is my height, but it was 20 pounds heavier than I had ever been prior to these events.

The next year, in 1999, my boyfriend and I were married. We found out we were expecting again in 2001; I was scared and excited all at the same time. The doctors were not too worried and believed this pregnancy would progress normally. At five weeks I started having some problems, spotting and a little pain. They decided to do an ultrasound to see if they could find anything wrong and they found that I had an ectopic (tubal) pregnancy. The only solution was to surgically remove the fetus growing inside my fallopian tube. Luckily, they were able to save my tube, but we did have to mourn the loss of our baby. It was very hard, but I was also very determined to have a baby, so three months later I was pregnant again. What could go wrong this time? The doctors kept a much closer watch, and at eight weeks we saw a heartbeat and a peanut. We were ecstatic. My pregnancy went well, and my beautiful son, Tyler, was born on his due date.

After Tyler was born, life seemed to perk up for me a little. The only thing holding me back was the 25 extra pounds that I had kept of the 42 I had gained during my pregnancy. At this point I was about 156 pounds—pretty unhealthy for someone my height. Two years down the road, with my weight holding steady at 155 pounds, we found out we were expecting again. Unfortunately, at twelve weeks we learned that the baby had died, and I had to undergo another D & C and endure another loss. Imagine my state of mind. Why me? I thought. I didn't think I could handle more loss.

Then my determination kicked in, and four months later I was pregnant again.

I was very excited and *very* afraid. Nine months later, my baby girl, Tara Lyn, was born. I gained another 10 pounds during the pregnancy. At 164 pounds I was trying to deal with a three-year-old, a newborn, and depression. Eight months later, I was in the doctor's office bawling my eyes out about my weight and my problems. The doctor said, "Honey, I think you are suffering from postpartum depression." I thought, No way: I love being a mom, and my kids make me very happy. But I learned that has nothing to do with it. You can love your kids completely and still be depressed. The doctor started me on antidepressants, but I had to stop taking them, because they just made my vertigo worse. Then I thought, What if my depression never goes away?

Fortunately, help was closer than I realized. Three months later my brother Tony approached our family with this wonderful idea to lose weight together. I hated being fat and now, because of the pact we made to eat healthy, exercise, and help each other out, a little over a year later I am a trim 123.2 pounds and just ran a half marathon. *Never* in a million years did I think I would be the one running down the street after working all day and taking care of two kids at home, but I am and I love the new me. I am healthy, happy, and proud to say I did this with my family.

We have started helping people in our city lose weight, and I have a team of ten people who I am coaching. They are doing great. I learned from this process that everyone has something serious going on in their life and thinks their problem is the hardest one to overcome. That is exactly the way I felt. But take it from me, if you stand up, stop making excuses, and do something about your health, the problems will not disappear overnight, but you will learn to work through these difficult situations and eventually get stronger and happier. Don't give up—you can do it!

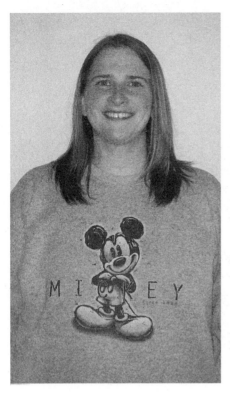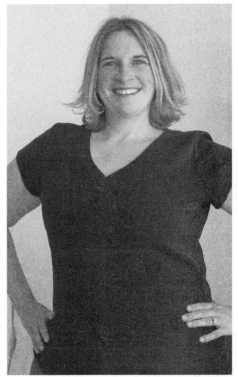

Jamie Sacks
Age at start of program: 29
Height: 5′4″
Starting weight: 298.0
Current weight: 197.8 (goal weight: 150)

As the test group for the F.A.S.T. diet, my family is about as diverse as a group of relatives could be. My sister Jamie, the entrepreneur, is very different from the others. Several years ago she became involved with Creative Memories, a wonderful organization that teaches people how to preserve their memories through scrapbooking. Jamie's Creative Memories business continues to grow, and it takes up much of her time. In spite of her work ethic and desire to be successful, Jamie had the most weight to lose. The human body is not meant to carry nearly 300 pounds on a small frame like hers.

In Jamie's defense, she faced the same problems that all fatties confront: poor diet role models, a busy lifestyle, two jobs, and (for women) extra weight after having children. The thing that was different about Jamie's situation was that . . . she was always fat. I can't remember a time when Jamie was thin, even as a child. Blame her genetics or whatever, but she has never been thin.

Because of our new video-game lifestyles and fast-food dinners in front of the TV, more and more children are starting life out overweight. As the years go on, overweight children become obese adults who never know what it feels like to be healthy, or thin. This is the hardest problem to overcome: if you have never been thin, then you probably have no idea how to eat properly and/or get thin. Most of all, you have no idea what being thin feels like, so how can you even know if you want to lose weight?

What makes Jamie's story so inspiring is her determination: when it comes to exercising, no one works harder. Once she had committed to the F.A.S.T. program, she would go to the gym at 11:30 p.m. if that was the only free time she had in the day. In spite of her weight and awkward shape (hips and a backside that are not proportional to the rest of her body), she would always work past her limitations and find a way to persevere.

If being more than twice her recommended weight were not enough of a challenge, Jamie also has bad knees. She occasionally would have to get cortisone shots because of the pain. Sometimes she would call me and say, "Tony, I don't know what to do for my workout today because I can't walk." But Jamie refused to quit. She never said, "I can't do it." Instead of letting down both the team and herself, she would always ask for help.

At first it was hard to figure out what she could and could not do at the gym. Her knee problems kept her off 75 percent of the equipment, and she could only use a machine for a short time. We asked her doctor a lot of questions. Through experimentation we eventually built a list of exercises that she could tolerate and do well. As the weight started to come off, her knees kept getting better, because they weren't carrying such a heavy load.

When our family started the F.A.S.T. diet, Jamie was on another plan. I pleaded with her to drop it, but she wouldn't. Finally, after she saw how much weight everyone else was losing, I was able to convince her to join us, and the results were fantastic. Eleven weeks later, I compared her weight loss to the previous eleven weeks when she had been on a different plan: she was losing slightly more than two times the weight while eating *more*.

Like many people, Jamie has a genetic predisposition and a physical disability that make it easy for her to be heavy. In many cases, both problems can be overcome. If you are someone who has always been big, then I have news for you: life is wonderful, but it is not always fair, and you are going to have to work twice as hard to lose half as much as everyone else. But the rewards are worth it. Although Jamie still has about 50 pounds to lose as of this writing, she has already lost more than 100 pounds. She can now climb, run, and wrestle with her children at the playground instead of standing on the sidelines watching. Even though she knows she will never have a supermodel's body, she realizes that it is important to have a long and healthy future ahead of her to spend with her children and loved ones.

No matter what exercise program you are on, you must use your doctor as a resource. All of them recommend that you check with your doctor before starting; however, we called our doctors not just to ask for permission but to gather information.

If you ask your doctor, "Can I work out at the gym?" he or she will say yes or no. You will learn far more if you say, "I really want to get healthy. If you had my disability, what exercises would you do? How would you do them? How long would you do them? How many times a week would you do them? How much weight would you recommend losing? Are there other things I could be doing? Should I stretch before I begin?" Ask, ask, ask! Doctors go through a lot of education and training so that they can wear those white coats. Doctors are smart. It is time for you to benefit from their knowledge.

If Jamie had never done the F.A.S.T. diet, she would have had no choice but to resign herself to the fact that she was just too fat to work out, and she would probably be 350 pounds instead of 197.8 pounds. Because Jamie never gave up, her goal weight of 150 is within sight.

Jamie is a born leader. If everyone had her work ethic and determination, more people would find the success they are looking for. From Jamie we learn that even though life is not always fair, you can *never* give up.

Jamie Sacks

I have been trying to lose weight since I was a teenager. I always remember myself as being a larger kid. When I look back at pictures of myself at a normal size, when I was eight and younger, I don't remember those times, but when I see pictures of me from age 10 and up, I remember everything. It is almost as if being heavy has been a part of me for so long that I have no recollection that there was a time when I was average.

I never had self-esteem issues about my weight because my mom always told me that I was a beautiful person and that if people didn't like me for who I was then they were not true friends. Now when I look back, that wasn't necessarily a good thing: I never saw what was so bad about being heavy until it was really hard to lose the weight.

After high school I tried many diets and none really worked. When I was engaged to be married, I joined Weight Watchers. I was 280 pounds and wanted to lose weight to look gorgeous in my wedding dress. I successfully lost 40 pounds, and I did look beautiful. Once I was married and the goal to fit in the dress was gone, my motivation disappeared, and unfortunately I had not learned anything that would help me keep the weight off. Over the course of two years, while I was trying to get pregnant, I gained those 40 pounds back and then some. I went to the doctor to discuss why I was having problems getting pregnant, and he said that my weight (298 pounds) was an issue.

I realized that one day I would have children (even though we were struggling now), and when it did happen, I did not want to be the mom who would have to say no when her kids asked, "Mom, will you play with me?" I was not going to be the mom who sat on the park bench because she was too tired and couldn't physically get up to play with her children.

Time passed, and in spite of my weight we were fortunate enough to have two babies, but I still had not taken any action to solve my weight problem. I was starting to feel like that tired mom I had never wanted to be. So I changed my eating habits, got some good advice about food, and started losing weight on my own. Like all the other times I tried, I was having some success and had lost some weight. Then my brother Tony suggested that our family lose weight together. I thought it was a phenomenal idea and was very excited when he shared it with us right before Thanksgiving. Everyone was thrilled with the idea of having such a strong support system to make this life change, so we all decided to go for it.

After some discussion, Tony and I decided that I would stick with what I was doing for a while since I had had some success and just incorporate the F.A.S.T. diet into what I was currently doing. That meant working out seven days a week and being involved in the accountability concept of daily check-ins with your team. I noticed that I just wasn't losing as much weight as the rest of the family. So I decided to count the calories I had been eating to see if I was close to the 1,250 I was supposed to be eating on the F.A.S.T. diet. I found that I was eating under 1,000 calories a day! I was not eating enough. After some serious thought, Tony and I decided that it would be best if I stopped dieting my own way and instead work on weight loss with the family. This was a really hard decision for me, because when you have something that is working you hate to give it up. It almost felt like I was starting over.

It turned out to be a great decision. In my first week, I lost 4.2 pounds, and my losses each week were double what I had been losing on my own. The F.A.S.T. diet has sparked a lifestyle change for me. I know I am not completely healthy, nor am I the size I want to be yet, but I do know that I am healthier than I was and I can fit into an XL shirt and size 18 pants (I used to be a size 28). The last time I fit into those pants was fifteen years ago!

Jeremy Dean

Age at start of program: 25
Height: 5'8"
Starting weight: 240.5
Current weight: 167 (goal weight)

Jeremy is my younger and only brother. When we started dieting, Jeremy seemed almost superhuman at times. He would lose 5 pounds one week and then 5 more the next. As we started to talk about what he was doing, I realized that Jeremy may have been the smartest of us all.

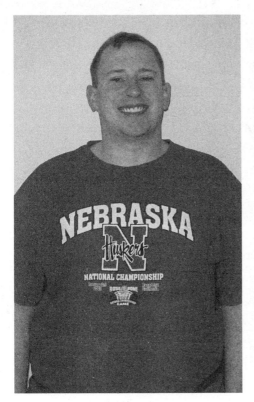 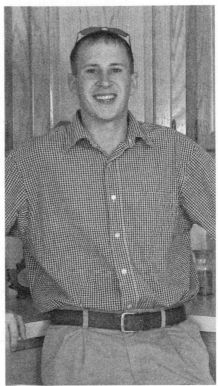

Jeremy was approaching 250 pounds at the beginning of this journey. Unlike the rest of the family, who had spent most of our lives heavy, Jeremy was a human yo-yo, swinging from 150 pounds to 225 six months later and then somehow back to 150 six months after that.

Whenever Jeremy was uncomfortable with his weight, he became a drastic dieter. He would eat almost nothing and literally starve himself. For a short time this approach would work, but we are all human and eventually, *we get hungry.* Once he broke his fast, he would quickly balloon up even bigger than before. This fluctuation is a very common but extremely unhealthy pattern for your body.

When we started the F.A.S.T. diet, Jeremy took a totally different approach to physical fitness than the rest of the family. This is
why he may have been the smartest of us all. Instead of grinding it
out every night at the gym, Jeremy decided to pick up a basketball.
He found an activity that he loved and pursued it with a passion.
For two hours every night Jeremy would play pickup basketball at
the gym. We estimated that he was burning 1,200 calories a day. It
is very hard to gain weight while exercising at that level, and Jeremy
was no exception. Even though he is short (like me) and can barely
touch the net on a basketball hoop, he loved it, and so he kept
doing it.

There are many ways to learn to love what you do while getting
healthy, and later in the process the activity actually becomes easier.
You learn what it feels like to feel good, and then you never want to
lose that feeling. But if you can find a sport or an activity that you
genuinely enjoy early on, you'll feel successful sooner. That's what
Jeremy did. He picked a sport that he loved and made sure it was
one that would make him sweat.

All you bowlers and golfers need to put away your bowling balls
and golf clubs. Although these forms of exercise are great to add to
your regimen after your regular workout, unfortunately, you simply
cannot exert yourself hard enough to work up a sweat doing them.
You never leave a bowling alley or a golf course smelling like a dead
rhino, and if you're not sweating, it's not a good workout (or at least it's
not challenging enough for you to lose much weight). Look for a more
demanding sport or activity that you'll come to love just as much.

Jeremy showed the rest of the family that working out can be
the most fun you can have. He was a role model for Tina, who soon
followed suit and discovered how much she loved to run. Now she
almost never goes to the gym, which she never liked all that much
anyway. She does what she loves—she runs.

Jeremy Dean

I had tried many different ways to lose weight in the last several years but didn't have any success. When my brother spoke to our family about doing a weight-loss program as a team, I was excited. I really liked the idea of counting on my family to help me. When you have a team like this, it makes losing weight a lot easier. For most people, it is the only way. One of my biggest fears was letting down my family. I sure don't like being the black sheep in the family or being the person who doesn't want something as bad as everyone else.

At my starting weight it took so much effort to walk up a set of stairs, play basketball, or do anything else aerobic. I also had severe joint pain. Now when I play basketball or run up stairs it doesn't even bother me. In five months I went from 240.5 to 177.2 pounds. I fought through the pain, the cravings, and everything else. The reason I kept pushing and pushing was to be the leader of the pack. There was simply no way I was going to be the one who let down the family.

People talk about their biggest fears in life being things like snakes or spiders. My biggest fear in life is not living up to the standards of my brother. It was very hard to grow up with four sisters and a brother who was ten years older than me. My brother has always been the toughest one in the family; he has no fear. I wanted to live up to that standard, and the F.A.S.T. diet was one way I could do it. I could show my brother that I was 100 percent committed to this program. Later, I realized that my success was not about my brother at all. It was about finding a way to hold myself accountable. Most people have someone in their life whom they look up to. If you were to make that person your partner and lose weight together, you would probably find, like I did, that it will drive you to succeed each day. It will get you off the couch on those days when you don't want to go to the gym. This accountability worked very well for me, and I was one of the first to lose my weight and reach my goal. I lost 70 pounds in about five months.

I know many people who are amazed by what we have accomplished. Now more than anything, I love helping others accomplish their goals. The hardest thing for most people is getting started. If you get on this program for two weeks and really work at it, you will see big results followed by a sense of accomplishment that will push you constantly to keep going when things get hard. There is no way I am going back to the old me.

This program is not just about eating right and exercising; it is about finding the support necessary to do them consistently. Every time I felt like cheating or quitting my family would push me just enough to keep me going.

Your team can do the same for you.

Julie Dean
Age at start of program: 24
Height: 5′0″
Starting weight: 226.5
Current weight: 158.8 (goal weight: 130.0)

Of all the strong women in my family, Julie is definitely one of the strongest. She is also the boldest: she has a mind of her own and will not hesitate to tell you what's on it. She is fun, wild, and a little crazy all mixed into one package. She is the first one on the dance floor and the last one to leave it. What is especially astounding about Julie is that she really does love who she is. Sure, she would like to have a big house and a little more money, but she honestly could be as happy at 250 pounds as she could be at 125.

Julie is also a single mother. In 2005 she and her boyfriend had a falling out, but not before she got pregnant. When we started the

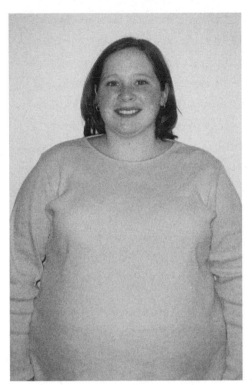 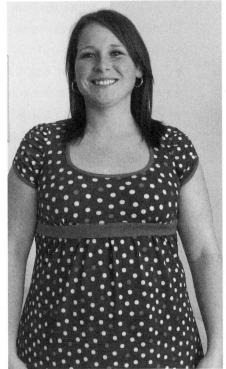

F.A.S.T. diet, Julie was in her seventh month. Talk about an obstacle! Well, as I've said before, "Find a way!" She did, and she did it the right way. She asked her doctor, "What can I do? How should I do it?" The doctor gave her some pregnancy exercises, and she was able to jump right into the program.

When her daughter, Kylin, was born, Julie had to face many new challenges. She had to work full-time while caring for a new baby and dealing with all the other responsibilities that come with being an adult. She realized right away that she was going to have to make some adjustments if she was going to stay on the F.A.S.T. diet. The family was already losing weight every week, and Julie had made a commitment to the team that she was not going to break.

First, she made plans to live with my parents for a while. Second, she waited until the baby went to sleep at night before working out. Sounds simple, doesn't it? Well, it really isn't. Most people have the same schedule: work all day, come home, eat, get the kids to bed, and then finally rest for a minute or two. Julie turned that minute or two into an hour and applied it to her health. From Julie we learn that you can follow the program even if you are raising a child on your own. And what better gift to give your child than a healthy parent?

Because Julie was exercising during her pregnancy, she only gained 21 pounds. She has always been pretty, but now, without the extra weight and with the added confidence, she is absolutely beautiful. You really never know what is under all that fat until you start taking it off. The real you is in there!

Julie Dean

My whole life I always thought that I wasn't really fat, I just had baby fat. I remember my mom putting a bikini on me when I was about ten years old and how my chubby belly was hanging over the little bottoms. I remember thinking, I don't think I should go out in public like this, but I kept reminding myself that it was just baby fat—it would go away. All through elementary school I was the chubby girl; I actually think I was wearing plus-size clothes by the time I was a sixth grader. When I hit junior high, I still had not gotten rid of the baby fat. I couldn't believe that it had stayed with me. I was stunned, yet I still didn't do anything about it. Junior high was hard for me; people started to get mean and judgmental, but it was nothing compared to the judgment I was about to encounter in high school.

I'll never forget my junior year of high school: I was seventeen, five feet tall, and nearly 200 pounds, and a football player who always hounded me told me to call Jenny Craig. At that moment, not only did I want to bawl my eyes out, I actually wanted to pick up the phone and call Jenny Craig. But I'm sure at that point I just ate another doughnut instead and felt sorry for myself. Maybe if I had stopped feeling sorry for myself I would have learned what I know now and my life would be so much different. I think I hoped a weight-loss fairy would sprinkle some fairy dust on my head and magically the weight would be gone. It didn't happen. So I just sat in the background, eating my high-calorie foods and slowly gaining more weight.

During the summer before my senior year in high school, I decided that I was going to go back in the fall looking like a fox. I would show them. I decided to start eating a no-carbs diet: Atkins. The first day I ate meat and cheese and drank lots of water and diet caffeine-free pop. The second day I ate meat and cheese and drank lots of water and diet caffeine-free pop. The third day was the same and so were the fourth, fifth, and sixth days. In a few months, I had lost 50 pounds and I felt great. I couldn't wait to start school again and show off the new me. On the first day of school, I wore the outfit that made me look the skinniest and everyone kept telling me how great I looked! I looked great, I felt great, and then . . . the lunch bell rang. Hmm . . . what should I have? How about pizza and French fries, a meal loaded with carbs. By the time I graduated from high school I had gained all the weight back and then some!

After graduation I worked in an office on a computer all day long. By the time I got home, I was so tired I just went to bed. After a few years I decided to try the no-carbs diet again. This time would be different; I wouldn't let myself gain the weight back. I lost the weight again but quickly gained it back plus a few extra pounds. I felt hopeless.

In June 2005, when I was twenty-four years old, I found out I was pregnant. I was thrilled but very scared. Not only was I already overweight, but I was going to gain more. At my first doctor visit, I weighed in at 201 pounds. Boy, was I feeling bad about myself that day. The doctor told me that I needed to start eating healthier so that my total weight gain would be between 25 and 30 pounds. My whole life I thought Big Macs were healthy, so do you think I got it when he told me to "eat healthier"? NO! Over the next few months I gained only a few pounds but then in one month I gained 10. I was shocked. I didn't know it at the time, but the 2,000 calories of Mountain Dew that I was drinking a day, plus all the food I was ingesting, added up to a hefty weight gain. By the time I was seven months pregnant, I was enormous: I had already gained 25.3 pounds with two months to go.

Then my life changed forever when my fabulous brother Tony said we were really going to do the diet we had talked about months before. The first thing I did was talk to my doctor to find out the limits for a pregnant woman who was overweight and had never exercised. How many calories should I eat a day? What exercises were safe for me? How often could I work out? The doctor told me to eat no less than 1,800 calories a day, and that I could work out five days a week but not on anything that I could easily fall off like a treadmill or a cross-trainer. I started by doing some light walking around the gym and then began doing a water aerobics class for an hour three times a week. Every day I told my assigned buddy how many glasses of water I drank, the amount of calories I ate for the day, how many calories I burned during exercise, and how much fiber I had. Finally, after one week of eating better, working out, and checking in every day with my partner, it was time for our first weigh-in. I didn't feel much lighter, but I had more energy and actually felt good. The anticipation was killing me: I stepped on the scale and my weight was 215 pounds! What? I'd lost 11 pounds! I was so excited I couldn't believe it! I think that week my family lost a total of 75 pounds. It was so motivating to see the people I love around me losing huge numbers just like me.

At the next weigh-in everyone lost just a pound or two each. Because we were expecting to lose double-digit pounds again and didn't, everyone felt a little down. We didn't realize that our bodies were in shock that first week. However, we didn't lose sight of our final goal, to lose weight and keep it off. Week by week I lost a pound or two.

Toward the end of my pregnancy, I started to gain a little weight back, which was normal. I continued to work out and eat right. Four weeks away from giving birth, I started Lamaze classes. During the second or third class we sat down on the floor to practice our breathing. Once we were done practicing, I remember jumping up and helping my boyfriend get up. I looked around and all of the other pregnant women in my class were holding their backs and moaning as their husbands or boyfriends slowly helped them off the floor. I thought, Wow, if it had not been for this wonderful idea my brother had to get our family healthy, I would be one of those women, feeling sorry for myself and holding my aching back and moaning. But instead I was full of energy and feeling great.

When I was thirty-seven weeks pregnant, I fell down a flight of stairs and sprained my ankle. I couldn't walk, and this made it very difficult—but not impossible—to exercise. I continued to eat right, and five times a week I would pick up a couple cans of vegetables and lift them like weights. This seems silly, I know, but it kept me in the game. Finally on February 21, 2006, my labor was induced. Your labor is supposed to be much easier when you exercise, and I believe it's true. My daughter was nowhere near ready to be born. I was not dilated at all, and she was head down, but her head was not engaged. My labor from start to finish was six hours and fifty-nine minutes; the doctors and nurses were surprised, because first-time moms are usually in labor for a minimum of twelve hours. Had I not trained my body, I could have been in labor for more than a day.

So now I am a new mom, with many new worries and about ten times busier than I could have ever imagined. Her father and I split up, so as a single mom with an infant, I try to manage my life so that I can continue to exercise every day and eat right. At first it was tough. I really struggled to get back to the gym every day, not because it was physically hard but because I had to find a babysitter. This is how the F.A.S.T. program really helped me: everyone knew I had to go to the gym, so people started offering to watch my daughter for an hour or two while I exercised. My sister and I took turns babysitting our kids. My teammates were pitching in, and we were all helping each other out.

Now my daughter is a year old, and I have a great routine: I work full-time while my mom watches her during the day. I come home at five and spend the next two to three hours playing with, bathing, and feeding my daughter. When she goes to bed, one of my parents watches her while I head off to the gym between 8:00 and 10:00 p.m. Some days, after my daughter goes to bed, I want to just crawl into bed and forget about the gym, but I know that my mom or another teammate would wonder why I hadn't gone to the gym and would hold me accountable.

I have lost a total of 67.7 pounds, with 28.8 to go. But this time is different; I have learned that I must change my lifestyle, not just what I eat. I am excited to see myself slim and trim and for my daughter to know a healthy mommy. I will pass what I have learned on to my daughter and future children. And now that our family has come together and made this program work, I know that my children will hold my grandchildren accountable as well.

The first thing we each had to overcome was years of making excuses and memories of our past diet failures. I call this diet baggage, and now I am going to help you get past yours.

Chapter 3

YOU CAN DO IT: DITCHING YOUR DIET BAGGAGE

B efore my family started the F.A.S.T. program, each of us had failed so many times at dieting that it was hard to believe that we could be successful even with the perfect program. Memories of past failures often destroy even the most well-meaning and motivated dieters. Before I teach you about food and exercise, let's tackle the baggage and excuses so that they don't sabotage your efforts.

The desire to be thin is such a phenomenon that almost everyone has tried to lose weight and failed. You know how it goes. Someone tells you about the new North Desert diet. All you eat is steak and chocolate. You think, Great . . . I love steak and chocolate. You start eating exactly along the guidelines of the program and before you know it you start to lose a little weight, maybe 10 or even 15 pounds. Life is good.

Then something happens. Things get really stressful at work

because of some big project or long hours. Your kids start driving you nuts. And there it is, that piece of pie in the fridge—and as luck would have it, it's not chocolate. You eat the piece of pie and your diet is ruined. For the next couple of months you take a one-day-on, one-day-off approach to the diet, but because you're never consistent again, you gain all the weight back—plus a few more pounds for the effort.

Three months later, you feel like a fatty and a failure again. You hear about a new diet pill, so you buy it and start all over. Over time, these failures add up to create what I call diet baggage. Diet baggage is a heavy emotional weight that you carry around with you. Every time you decide to get healthy, or are already dieting and thinking about cheating, you feel the weight of that baggage, and it is usually just enough negative energy to convince you to do the wrong thing.

It doesn't take much negativity to bring you down: "This is too hard" or "I don't feel like exercising today" or "I knew this wouldn't work!" or, worst of all, "I'm too old."

FORGIVE YOURSELF

It is time to let go of all that negative energy. It is time to forgive yourself for all the mistakes you made and empty promises you broke in the past. It is time to say, "I forgive me."

I cannot tell you how powerful it is to forgive someone else, but forgiving yourself is ... divine. I didn't understand this concept before I started this program, but now it is one of my core truths. We are so hard on ourselves that many times we sabotage our own best interests, refusing to forgive ourselves when we would readily forgive someone else. If you are going to achieve your goal of being the healthiest you can be, you must break this habit.

Forgive yourself! Forgive yourself! Forgive yourself!

Take a few minutes alone. Drive out to the country for a few hours or shut yourself in a private room where no one will bother you. Then go over in your mind every painful memory of a weight-loss attempt that failed and forgive yourself once and for all. Just let it go. When your life is over, you won't get points for feeling bad or putting yourself down. Human life is priceless and everyone has the potential for greatness.

Seemingly ordinary people can do great work and accomplish great things. Consider J. K. Rowling, the author of the Harry Potter books. Once dead broke, she is now worth a billion dollars. Imagine if she had been too busy to pick up a pen and write: the world would be a less joyful place. She makes us think by stretching our imaginations. She does the kind of good that we need more of in this world.

Maybe you have an unknown talent as well, but because of your failed attempts to become healthy you start to doubt your dream. So you never pick up the pen or the paintbrush or take the helm of a sailboat or put on those downhill skis. Being overweight and out of shape prevents you from doing what you really want to do. It steals not only your energy but also your self-confidence.

Most of us spend a lifetime complaining about the things we don't have instead of being grateful for what we do have. We constantly think, speak, and act out the words of failure because we have made mistakes. Beating ourselves up for things we can't change in the past has a huge effect on our future. If you are going to get over your past failures and live to your full potential, you will first need to forgive yourself. You only have one life to live. Take the time to heal your inside, and I will show you how to heal your outside. It really is as simple as saying "I forgive me!" and believing it.

You are reading this book because you want something *better* for yourself. You have settled for less than you think you are worth, and you want help to find the real you. But you will never find that person unless you give yourself a chance to succeed. *I* forgive you, so now you should do the same. *Forgive yourself.*

Forgiving yourself is the first step. If you want to lose weight consistently (and I know you do), you must drastically change the way you think about what is possible and what you are capable of doing.

FOCUSING ON POSSIBILITIES
INSTEAD OF IMPOSSIBILITIES

When my parents started going to the gym (which they did only after getting the go-ahead from their doctors), their first workouts were horrifying. I supervised them closely as each walked on the treadmill for thirty minutes at 1.3 to 1.8 speed with no incline; that is a *very* slow pace—about a third of the speed at which a healthy person could walk up a hill backwards. A ninety-year-old woman could push a walker faster.

Being even a little bit active was such a shock to their systems that both of them almost fell: I had to hold my mother's hands and then my father's as each stepped down the six inches from treadmill to floor. The experience was so uncomfortable for my parents that they would have quit the very minor workout I devised for them before they even started if I had not been there.

The truth is that their minds did not want them to change, and that's true for your mind, too. The human mind will invent excuses to make you lazy . . . until you get healthy. Then your mind does everything it can to convince you to stay healthy. You should see

my parents now: it's almost hard to believe they are the same people. My dad walks on the treadmill at the highest incline of 15 at a
4.4 pace for an hour. He does this extremely rigorous workout regularly. My mom ran and finished a one-mile race. This is a woman
who, in the last thirty years, has never run more than three steps in
any direction. In the past she wouldn't have been able to run a mile
even if a lion was chasing her.

OVERCOME YOUR EXCUSES

Have you ever made an excuse to not eat right or work out? We all
have. We make excuses for everything. Sometimes I will make an
excuse for why I don't have to eat right or exercise that day, and at
that exact moment I think, I am right as to why I don't have to do
this. Then, once I start to think logically, I realize that I'm not right;
I'm simply making excuses.

When my family started this program, everyone agreed that he
or she would work out every day, without exception. There would
be only one exception: I told them, "If your doctor says you cannot
work out, then you can't. But unless a doctor tells you to stop, keep
working out."

Don't hesitate to call your doctor for advice. For example, if
you come down with the flu and have been working out every
day for the past thirty days, tell your doctor, "I really need to do
some exercise today that will not make my flu worse. What would
you recommend?" If your doctor tells you to stay in bed, then
enjoy a well-earned rest. But it's likely he or she will say, "Well, a
casual walk around the block for twenty minutes won't hurt you."
And then that is what you must do. Find a way to get past your
excuses.

I'm not suggesting that you become a workout fanatic. Rather, I want you to make an iron-clad commitment to exercise and eat right every day, no matter what. There are a few things we all will commit to doing no matter what (and they are often for other people). For example, if you need to pick up your kids from school at a certain time, you make sure you are there *no matter what.* You will move work and cancel all kinds of activities to make sure you don't leave your kids stranded. Well, I believe that your exercise routine needs to be one of those "must-do" items that is always on your list and that you find a way to do *no matter what.*

I told my family, "If you are in a car wreck and find yourself in bed in a body cast from head to toe and the only thing sticking out of the cast is one finger, your exercise for the day would be to bend that finger back and forth for thirty minutes." It sounds extreme, but that is how committed you have to be. Remember, we are talking about your health, and without your health you have nothing. It's okay to get a little extreme.

If I told you that I would give you $10 million if you worked out for an hour a day for the next 365 days, would you do it? Of course you would, and you wouldn't skip a single day, even if it meant working out late at night or before dawn. That is the attitude you need to have to succeed on the F.A.S.T. diet. As a mentor of mine once told me, "Exceptions are the enemy of excellence."

Anything that prevents you from exercising or eating right is an excuse. Here are a few of the most common:

Busy Lifestyle

"But I just have so much going on right now" is everyone's favorite excuse to avoid exercising and eating right. To make it worse, everyone thinks he or she is the only one in the world who is short on time. This phrase comes in many shapes and sizes: "I am going to start exercising right after the holidays, when I'm not so busy" or "I just got a promotion and need to spend more time at the office, but I'll start exercising again when things have settled down." But the fact is, almost everyone has a lot going on and feels too busy to put time aside to be active. It is just the way we are wired. Even so, we have to see this phrase for what it is—an excuse.

If you think about it, you'll see that there is no advantage to postponing your exercise program. Let's assume that after the holidays you actually did start working out and kept it up all year. At about the same time next year you will be at the peak of health. You will have learned all the skills to be healthy, and you will never go back to being a fatty. Are you really going to dump all that knowledge and start eating like a pig again around the holidays? *No!* Once you realize how good you feel, both physically and mentally, you won't be able to imagine going back to your old habits.

What we are really talking about here are priorities, plain and simple. If you are going to be healthy, you will need to plan your life around your fitness goals, not the other way around. That is the only way it can work. You cannot be successful and healthy by fitting exercise in when you have nothing else to do. It never works when you do it that way, because you will never find the time.

I believe that if you lose everything in your life except your health, you can still do great things. If you lost every dollar you have, your spouse, parents, and even the family dog, but you still had your health, you could recover. It would be possible to get your life back. You could work ninety hours a week, find new love, build new relationships. There would be hope.

But without your health, you have nothing! Your health must come first, so plan your life around it. After all, we are only talking about an hour or ninety minutes a day. How much time do you spend watching TV a day? Or chatting on the phone with friends? Or lounging with a cup of coffee, reading the paper? I'll bet at least that much. Why don't you read the paper at the gym instead? Or check out a good book on CD at your local library and listen to it while you work out? If you took the next year and exercised every day for an hour while listening to language tapes, you could learn a new language and get healthy at the same time.

Later I will show you how to build your team, and you will probably use excuses to convince your team why you can't work out on a particular day. The team must become the master and not a slave to excuses.

Ill Health

Health issues—"I broke my leg" or "I have the flu" or "I suffer from migraines." These are good excuses, right? Wrong!

If you have a broken leg, you still have to eat properly, right? I am not a physiotherapist, but even I know that a broken leg can't stop you from eating healthy foods and staying below your maximum calorie intake. What about exercise, though? All cardio exercises use your legs, right? Wrong! Many exercise machines are designed to work only the arm muscles, and I bet that your doctor will encourage you to use them for an hour a day if you are able to get to the gym. Learn to think beyond limiting excuses. Is your health issue a valid reason not to work out? Ask your doctor.

Tight Budget

"But what if I can't afford a gym membership?" you say. Try asking yourself this question instead: "How can I afford to go to the gym?" When you phrase the question this way, you engage your mind to come up with solutions. When you ask the question using the word *can't,* your mind just shuts down.

When my family first started going to the gym, I charged my parents' membership on my credit card, and one of my sisters signed up through a program at her job. Tracy bought used exercise equipment. Once we had decided we were going to work out, we found a way. You need to do the same thing: call a small gym and ask about specials.

But let's say you have exhausted every option, and you really can't afford a gym membership. I have great news for you—you have legs! And it is likely that you live in the world. As luck would have it, the world is huge. I'm not a trainer, but I believe almost anyone with legs can learn to power walk or even run. Start slow and go a little farther every day. *Overcome! Find a way!* Be creative to find solutions. Once again, if I told you I would give you $10 million to find a way to exercise every day even without a gym membership, you would. There is no way you would say, "I just can't figure it out." You'd find a way.

Excuses Other People Make For You

There is another kind of excuse that you won't even make, but it will affect you nonetheless: the excuses other people make for you. These are the most deadly of all. I once heard that 90 percent of people don't care if you are hurt or upset and the other 10 percent are happy about it. This may or may not be true, but unless the people talking to you about your diet or workouts are doctors or teammates, ignore them completely. Everyone has something to say, but most people have no clue what they are talking about, especially when it comes to health and weight loss.

A person may try to deliberately undermine your progress with excuses like "You can miss one day—it won't kill you. I never get to see you anymore." You feel so guilty that you agree and buy into the excuse, thereby putting his or her feelings first and undermining your own health. The sad truth is that the changes you're making in your life may threaten other people. They may be jealous or just want to restore the comfortable, predictable routine.

In some cases, the sabotage isn't even deliberate. Say you are about to go to the gym, when you meet a friend who says, "Did you hear about Joe? He lost fifty pounds eating a low-carb diet." Suddenly you wonder if you should be eating less carbs, too, so you do. Without carbs, your body starts losing energy and you feel lethargic and always hungry. Then you start to eat a little more and exercise a little less and pretty soon you are a fatty again. Ignore advice you hear on TV or from anyone who is not on your team and maintain your focus on the F.A.S.T. plan. (But *always* listen to your doctor.)

Are you ready to ditch your diet baggage? Good. Do you refuse to play the excuse game? Great. Are you going to exercise and eat right every single day, except when your doctor tells you not to? Excellent! Your outlook is nearly perfect.

Tomorrow Never Comes

When you diet, you often have many good days in a row and then suddenly a bad day. As soon as the bad day happens, you think, Tomorrow I will get back on the wagon. Tomorrow I will eat right and exercise really hard. In fact, tomorrow I am not going to eat at all, and I will exercise two hours instead of thirty minutes. Actually, tomorrow I will skip work and exercise all day.

That's right, eight hours of exercise and all I will eat is one banana and some tofu.

Then, of course, tomorrow comes and the first thing you eat is a doughnut and a bowl of ice cream and then you preorder a pizza to be delivered at exactly noon so you can start scarfing it down the second your lunch hour starts.

Ladies and gentlemen, here is the truth: tomorrow never comes.

No matter what you do, it is still always *today*. You can't do anything about tomorrow and you can't do anything about yesterday, but you can have an immediate impact right now. So if you fall off the wagon, don't let your mind trick you into starting anything tomorrow, next week, or when the new year starts, because the only thing you can control is *now*. Next time you slip, get right back up, dust yourself off, and congratulate yourself for not waiting until tomorrow.

One of my favorite advertisements was for a place that sold crabs in Dallas, Texas. The side of the building was painted into a big bulletin board that said FREE CRABS TOMORROW! The sign was there every day and let me assure you, no one ever got free crabs. Take charge today!

BEWARE OF THE FOOD REWARD PROGRAM

All right then, how is your brain? A little mushy? Feeling good? Here is the last piece of brain food for you. It is called the *food reward program*. Someone will start on our program, or any other diet, and instantly succeed by losing 10 or 15 pounds. They stand on the scale, and lo and behold, they just broke the 20-pound mark. Everyone is screaming and yelling, "Way to go, Mary! Wow, you look so good; you are doing great." On the way home Mary thinks, Yeah, I am doing great. I am so proud of myself; I need to reward myself for all my efforts. I think tonight, but just tonight, I am going to not track my calories and eat whatever I want. I have done so well I think I might just not exercise tomorrow.

When this moment comes for you, Mary's thinking will make total sense: like Mary, you deserve to be rewarded for your efforts, and more food and less exercise should be that reward. *This is crazy!* If you stop and think rationally for ten seconds, you will quickly realize that your brain is playing a trick on you to get you to go back to your old habits. Get it? No? Then let me use a different but similar context to get my point across.

Imagine that your girlfriend is an alcoholic. For years you have been trying to intervene and help her, but to no avail. Finally, her family gets together and does an intervention. Suddenly, your girlfriend is receptive: if all of her loved ones are concerned, certainly they can't all be wrong.

Your girlfriend stops drinking. She hasn't touched alcohol for weeks, and she is very proud of her efforts. When a person accomplishes something, it only makes sense to celebrate, right? So tell me, would you take her out for a drink to celebrate her sobriety? That's crazy, right? So why would you celebrate your weight loss with food? Still not clear? Here's another scenario.

Your brother has a drug problem. He is a heroin junkie, and many times you've walked into the house and found him passed out on the floor with a needle sticking out of his arm. Your family steps in, and before you know it three months have passed and your brother is drug free. Would you say, "Hey, Jimmy, congratulations on being drug free for three months. Let's shoot up to celebrate." That's crazy. You don't celebrate not doing drugs by shooting up, you don't celebrate sobriety with a few beers, and you should never celebrate dieting success with food. It simply doesn't make sense, and it *never* makes you feel better.

Remember

- Forgive yourself.
- Don't make excuses.
- Take charge today.
- Celebrate your successes—but not with food.

Now that you're in the right frame of mind to begin the F.A.S.T. program, it is time to create your team.

Chapter 4

CREATING YOUR TEAM: LOGISTICS AND PITFALLS

I have no idea why it took me so long to figure out the team concept, because our team was already in place. Once we were up and running, it was clear that we should have been doing this all along. All we needed was someone to step up and say, "Hey, let's work together. How could it possibly make sense to lose weight alone when we have each other?" As soon as I got up the nerve to do that, my family immediately rallied behind the idea and the rest is history.

I now know that for most people it is not quite that easy. Not everyone has a family like ours or a group of friends who are all overweight and want to get healthy. I didn't realize this until we started to get media attention. Reporters would always ask, "What is the secret to your diet?" Without any hesitation, one of my sisters would step forward and say, "Without a doubt, I think our family was the key. Without them, there is no way we could have succeeded." The first time this happened, the reporter's reaction surprised me: by the look on her face you would have thought we'd just told her that her kids were ugly and her husband was a fool. She responded in a mean voice, "Well, not everyone has a family like yours." What is your problem? I thought and then just shrugged it off until the same thing happened again and again.

Once I started thinking about it and realized they were all exactly right, I decided that a team didn't have to be an actual family: it could be your coworkers, your friends, your neighbors, or any group who wanted to unite to reach the common goal of losing weight and getting healthy. I wanted to prove that anyone who really wanted to lose weight could start a team.

This revelation was so important because without a team most people cannot diet successfully. There is magic in the team. Forming a support group of like-minded people with the same goal creates synergy. Suddenly, you are no longer one person fighting against the world and all the food in it; instead, you are an army fighting to win as a group. When one person has a bad day, the others jump in to reassure, "You can do it!" The power of support is astounding. Plus, the people who you spend most of your time with will be talking about the same things you are: your team and your diet.

"Hey, Joe, how many calories did you burn last night?"

"Actually, Mary, I broke the treadmill record—1,086 calories in one hour."

Your shared goals will quickly become your passion, and you'll be glad to have support so you will not have to face the challenge alone. You won't be able to wait for the chance to share a victory with your teammates. Your individual successes become motivation for the group, and the group's success becomes motivation for its members. I will say it again: the team is nothing short of magic.

People fail at dieting for one reason: they cheat one time. Those ten minutes of overeating or indulging cause them to quit dieting and maybe not try again for a year. Those ten minutes cost you, the dieter, a year and sometimes ten years. You may have been doing everything right, and because of ten minutes, you blow it for a whole year. With a team for support, those ten minutes will only last for . . . ten minutes. Then a teammate will step in and say, "C'mon, Jamie, you can do it." And instead of blowing it for the next year, you are instantly right back on track. Actually, you never get off track, because if you can recover from small slipups, then you are dieting the right way. The team helps us overcome the fact that we are all human and we will all make mistakes. Most of us make them all the time. That is why you must have a team.

RECRUIT YOUR TEAM

Early on in the F.A.S.T. program, a friend of mine who had expressed interest in the diet asked me, "How can I get involved?" I told him that I would be happy to help him if he could find a group of family members, friends, or coworkers who would join with him. He then asked the question that you are probably thinking right now, "What would I say to them?" How about, "Hey, Bill. You know, the other day I couldn't help but notice how fat you are. Do you want to start dieting with me?" or "Hey, Mary, how would you like to start dieting and exercising every day with no exceptions?" As you can see, no matter how you ask the question, it doesn't come off right and usually sounds insulting or intimidating.

I pondered this problem for several days, but I couldn't come up with a solution. Then it came to me: the answer was to not ask a question at all, but to pique the person's interest by telling a good story. After all, everyone loves a good story, and this one is great.

Here's how it works. Approach the person you are hoping to recruit and say, "Hey, did you see the story on *Good Morning America* about the family who lost five hundred pounds?"

Now really, is this going to offend anyone? No way. What this statement does is make someone curious.

"No, I didn't. Where are they from?"

"Omaha, Nebraska. This family of eight got together and lost 500 pounds in one year and then they helped a hundred more people lose 2,500 pounds. I'm reading their book right now, and it's so simple how they did it."

What someone is going to say right after that is, "How did they do it?"

Now look what you have done. In front of you is a captive audience just waiting to hear what you are going to say next. All you have to do is tell him or her a little about what you have read in the first few chapters of this book and then say, "The program is actually very simple and I was going to start it. Have you ever thought of doing something like this to get healthy?"

Next to no one will say, "No, not really. I enjoy having no clothes that fit and having people stare at me all the time because I am so obese. Oh, yeah, and I just love the fact that I don't fit in an airplane seat and have to buy two seats each time I fly." The usual response is "I might be interested."

Then you say, "Great. If I get a group together, I'll let you know. By the way, do you know anyone else who might be interested?"

"Well, yes, my husband might, and I work with two ladies who might want to join."

Believe me, pretty soon the people around you will start buzzing with the idea of creating a weight-loss team. "Hey, John, are you going to be on the team?" "What team?" "You mean you haven't heard? Well, let me tell you what Suzy is doing." Once people start hearing about this, they are interested. When we first started getting publicity, things got out of control for a while because we were always getting calls from news and radio people. Family, friends, and coworkers were also amazed and started asking how they could get involved. Although people are very hesitant to talk about their weight problems, they are not hesitant when a real solution pops up. Everyone who has a weight problem is looking for a solution. When someone comes along with a legitimate plan, they want to hear more.

I think this is the best way to recruit your team, but if the company you work for has a wellness coordinator, ask that person to help you get the word out. These people want to help and they honestly may not know what to do. Sure they know all about food and exercise, but remember, they were trained the old-fashioned way. The old-fashioned way of dieting was a solo program, which I truly believe doesn't work anymore. There is simply too much temptation, too many fast-food restaurants, and way too many vending machines.

Another approach is to send a letter or an e-mail to the people you want to recruit. I know the last thing you want to do is offend anyone, and a letter is very private: people can throw it away if they are offended or not interested without bringing attention to themselves. Here's a sample letter:

Dear Friend:

Last week I heard a story about a family of eight in the Midwest who lost 500 pounds in a year on a diet that lets them eat whatever food they want but teaches the secrets of motivation and moderation. I was shocked when I heard that all of them were successful, regardless of their work schedules, personal obstacles, or age. I decided to read their book and, to be honest, the program is easy. It contains very simple diet and exercise principles that most of us already know. Then we take that information and create a team to help us get through the rough spots.

Like most people, I have tried dieting several times and always failed. Usually I start out great and then I have a bad day because of stress at work or something else. Then that bad day torpedoes the whole diet. This book contains the solution for that bad-day problem.

The secret is to create a team of friends working together to help each other through those bad days. I have decided that I am going to create a small group to help me finally get in shape. We would create a support group that will help us do it together, instead of trying to do it alone and failing like I have so many times in the past.

The book tells you everything, including all the secrets they have used to have success. If this sounds interesting to you at all, please give me a call. If not, just ignore this letter. You are a good friend, and if I would want support from someone, it would be you.

If you send out twenty letters like this one to your friends and family, I guarantee you'll find enough people to form your group.

It really doesn't matter how you come up with your team. Just do it. Getting healthy is a process of taking steps that propel you toward your goal. At the same time, you need to unlearn all of the bad habits you picked up from the sales pitch on the back of a box of "fat-free" cookies.

For me, the bigger the team, the better. From a logistics standpoint, six to nine people is ideal, but if you're more ambitious and want to assemble a larger group, go for it. Ask your boss to send a memo to the whole company. Soon you will have all kinds of people working together and your group will be the only thing anyone is talking about.

When it comes to dieting, big groups are happy groups. So if you want to go big and you think you can do it, then do it. Make this a part of your life. I did and I have never regretted it for a second. It is an awesome thing to help yourself and, at the same time, help others.

ASSIGN TEAM TASKS

Now that the team is in place, what do you do next?

- Choose a record keeper. Someone needs to track each team member's current weight, height, age, calories needed to maintain weight, how many calories he or she currently eats, starting weight, and overall pounds (and percentage) lost. My family's chart looked like this:

| | Current | | | Calories to | | Currently | Starting | Overall | Total |
	Weight	Height	Age	Maintain	-500	Eats	Weight	% Lost	Pounds Lost
Men									
Dad	170.0	66	60	1,580	1,080	1,200	271.5	37.38%	101.5

It is important to carefully monitor these numbers. The record keeper will gather the starting weight, height, and age for each team member at the first weigh-in. This information will be used to calculate the number of calories each person should eat per day to first lose weight (the −500 column) and then maintain his or her weight loss. (I'll show you how to do the calculations in chapter 6.) At each weekly weigh-in, the record keeper will update the entries as needed.

- Pick the date, time, and location for the first weigh-in. Each week you will need to have a weigh-in, and it's easiest to do it at the same location every time. The home that hosts the weigh-ins must have a digital scale that registers to at least two-tenths (0.2) of a pound–198.6 pounds, for example. A scale that records to the half pound is not good enough, unless it is your only choice and you cannot afford to buy a new one; a scale that reads to a tenth of a pound is best. You want the weights to be precise because there will be some weeks when you lose only 0.2 pound. If your scale is not exact, it will round the weight off, and you'll seem to weigh the same as you did the previous week.

▪ Pick your first partner and decide on a check-in time each day. Exchange contact information (phone number, e-mail address, etc.). After your first weigh-in, call your partner every day to review how you're doing on the F.A.S.T. diet.

▪ Review the responsibilities of being part of the team:

• Hold your teammates accountable. Your teammates are not supposed to tell you what you *want* to hear; it's their responsibility to tell you what you *need* to hear.

• Help your teammates overcome any excuses or obstacles that prevent them from exercising or eating right (unless your advice contradicts a doctor's instructions).

• It is important to push your teammates toward their goals even when you can't push yourself.

• Avoid making judgments; for example, don't say that a teammate has a bad attitude just because he or she won't accept your excuses.

• Call a teammate and ask for help when you feel like you can't do it. Don't try to fight this battle alone.

• Consult a teammate before you cheat. Give him or her a chance to help you.

• Do not try to work exercise around your life; you must work your life around exercise, or you will never make it.

Commonly Asked Questions

What do I say to a teammate who is having a bad day and wants to overeat or has already started overeating?

Sometimes a simple "Come on, buddy, you can do it" is all you need. Often an attitude change will happen when a person thinks someone else cares. However, if a teammate is adamant about overeating and simply will not back down about cheating, then your approach must be as radical as his: get reinforcements, visit the teammate in crisis, and say over and over, "This is not just about you." Remember, if one person in your group fails, it will be easy for a second to follow, and soon everyone has become the spokesperson for Snickers. Only two things can happen when a person needs help. You push him to stay focused and he does or he quits. Either way you did your part. If you don't hold the person accountable and let him slide, then he'll quit after a few weeks of mediocre results. See, the only way to respond is to say and do whatever you can to hold them accountable.

What do I do if a teammate wants to quit?

First of all, no one who is losing weight ever quits, no matter how hard he or she is pushed. So if a teammate has hit a weight plateau or is gaining a few pounds and is talking about quitting, go to the gym with him or her. Do a thorough daily check-in. Plead with the person to finish out the week, because a successful weigh-in will keep the team intact.

What do I do if someone is disruptive?

Kick them out without hesitation. Your health is a serious issue. If someone was being disruptive to your family, your finances, or anything else important in your life, you would make a change to exclude them from these activities. Your health is your most valuable physical asset. If someone is disrupting the team's progress, raise your concerns with the group, and if everyone agrees, ask the person to leave. If they are going to be disruptive now, they will only get worse as things get more difficult.

FIRST TEAM PROJECTS

Now that you have assembled your team, and team members have committed to a time and place for weekly weigh-ins, exchanged contact information, chosen a partner, and agreed to check in with their partner every day once the F.A.S.T. diet has begun, it's time to get to work. Here are your first assignments:

- Weigh yourself. Knowing how much you weigh before you start dieting is a good idea. Some people actually lose a few pounds before the first official weigh-in!
- Start a diet log to keep track of your food and exercise throughout the F.A.S.T. program. At the back of this book is a thirty-day diet log to get you started. For three days before your first weigh-in, write down everything you eat and list any exercise you do. Don't change anything you normally do during these three days—just write it down as accurately as possible. (After the first weigh-in, when the F.A.S.T. diet officially starts, you'll track your food in order to stay within the parameters of the diet, but for now don't worry about the diet. Just keep track of what you're already doing.)

Keeping track of food and exercise is a critical element of the F.A.S.T. diet. It will make losing and maintaining weight easy. The next chapter shows you how to accurately keep track of what and how much you eat. You'll be a pro in just a few days.

Chapter 5

TRACKING FOOD: CARBS, FATS, AND CALORIES

First you need to learn how to keep track of what and how much you're eating in a diet log. There are thirty tracking pages at the back of this book where you'll record water, calories, fat, carbohydrates, fiber, protein, and any vitamins, supplements, or medications you take. It is important to get comfortable using these tracking pages right away (or create your own food journal to track the same items). You should keep your tracking pages with you as much as you can. Many people will try to write on scraps of paper when they start and then transfer the numbers when they get home. This never works. Your tracking pages are your friend; keep them with you.

People sometimes tell me that they don't want to count calories, but think about this for a minute. Do you count your money? Yes. Why? Because it has value. In fact, most people spend a lot of time keeping track of their money: how much they have, how much the average light bill is, how much they spend on telephone bills, and so on. But when it comes to our bodies we think it's okay to skimp. It takes just sixty seconds to write down what you ate at a meal and how much water you drank. Clearly, you are worth the small investment of time. Nothing is more important than your health.

Once you start to pay attention to what is going into your body, you'll begin to question your priorities. Let's say you own a car. You'll probably wash and wax it every week for five years until you sell it. But when it comes to your body, you barely have a clue about the junk you are putting inside it. Why? I think that we take our bodies for granted because we keep them for a lifetime.

Learning to count calories and track how much fat, protein, et cetera, you are eating is a lot like learning to type or learning to drive. At first everything seems cumbersome, but soon enough you get the hang of it and find that it takes little time or effort. In fact, just like typing or driving, counting calories becomes indispensable. When people reach their goal weight in the F.A.S.T. program, they are no longer required to track calories in a diet log, but almost everyone keeps on doing it. Tracking really does give you the control that you are craving. Life becomes easier and more enjoyable.

For the first several weeks, you will record the nutritional content by reading food labels and transferring that information into your log. At first this may take about thirty minutes a day, but it will seem like an hour. After about ten days, the whole process should take about five minutes a day.

Being vigilant about tracking your food will benefit you in two ways. First, you will lose weight consistently, because you know exactly how many calories you are eating and can gauge whether you are getting enough fiber and protein. As time passes, with this stored information about your eating habits at your fingertips, your diet journal will become a treasure map that will lead you to the big red X, which is your health. If you have a bad week, it will be a snap to look back and compare it with a good week; instead of guessing what the problem is, you will be able to pinpoint it precisely.

Some diets count points instead of calories. I think this is short-sighted: not all meals have points, but they all have calories. When you are counting points or using any other oversimplified way of tracking food, you lose focus on the other keys to eating a healthy diet. You never get the education you need about food when you are paying attention to the points.

Second, you'll learn a lot about your body and food when you count your calories, protein, fats, carbs, and fiber. You will learn what makes your body feel good and what makes it feel bad. You will learn which foods make you feel tired and which foods make you feel alive. For many people, eating high-fiber foods first thing in the morning really starts the day right. Others experience real lows around mid-day, and in the past they would have reached for a soda or a candy bar; now they eat fruit instead and notice how much better they feel.

Almost by accident, you become an expert on *you*. At a point in the F.A.S.T. diet, a light will switch on and you will suddenly think, I get it. I understand why I am overweight and I really know what needs to change so I don't have to stay this way. There is a unique kind of pride and confidence that comes with understanding your own body. Tracking your food will help you attain it.

HOW TO TRACK YOUR FOOD

Let's say that the first thing you eat for the day is an apple. At the back of this book is a list of Nutritional Values for Common Foods (page 181). Here are the values for a medium apple:

Food or Beverage	Serving Size	Calories	Fat (grams)	Carbs (grams)	Fiber (grams)	Protein (grams)
Apple, medium	1	81	0.5	21.1	3.7	0.3

Write these numbers in the appropriate columns in your log. Many of the foods we eat today will have a label that lists all the values you are looking for. Copy them into your log. In addition to the basic information we are tracking, these labels are very useful for determining sodium, sugar, cholesterol, and whether your food contains good or bad fats. Later on you can learn how these nutrients impact your body and your health.

Your next meal is something a little tougher to find: you really want to eat orange roughy fillets for lunch. Of course, you look in the back of this book and orange roughy is not listed; so what do you do? You have three choices. Option 1 is to guess: "After all, it's fish, and fish is good. I suppose this fillet would be about 150 calories." I bet you know how I feel about that. If you are ever going to be healthy, guessing is never the right answer; guessing is what you've been doing for all the years you've been getting fatter. Guessing, estimating, and approximating are all recipes for disaster when it comes to dieting. So don't choose door number 1. No guessing.

Option 2 is a much better choice. Look up the information in a nutritional-values book. Several good ones are listed in Resources (see page 247). Some of these books list as many as five thousand foods, and there are also digital versions that look like PDAs. If you own one of these books, you can quickly find all the numbers on just about anything you want to eat.

Option 3 is to use the Web, which provides extensive information on dieting and healthy eating. Type "calories in orange roughy" into any search engine and numerous sites will pop up with the information you need. My favorite is calorie-count.com. You should be able to get all the information on calories, protein, fat, carbs, and fiber from one site. If your site doesn't list protein or fiber, then don't use it and find another one.

If you can't find the complete nutritional information
for a food, then you can't eat it.

This rule is hard for some people because it involves breaking old habits. If someone hands you a piece of birthday cake, you eat it, right? Not on the F.A.S.T. diet. Unless you baked the cake yourself and can calculate the portion size and nutritional values (or the person who baked it can give them to you), or you copy the information from the package and cut yourself an appropriate-size portion, you can't eat it. It's that simple: if you can't get the numbers, don't eat the food. People who make exceptions to this rule fail.

Many situations will come up that will tempt you to do the wrong thing. Halloween is a great example. Those little candy bars are right in your face. You think, It's just a little candy bar, how many calories can it have? You pick it up to check the calories, but they're not listed. Then you remember that they were printed only on the big bag. So, if you can't find the big bag, you can't eat the individually wrapped candy. (By the way, some of those tiny candy bars have 150 calories each and are barely enough for one bite.) Don't make exceptions.

If your food or beverage doesn't have a label listing everything it contains, it is usually a good sign that the manufacturer doesn't want you to know because the food is filled with trans fats and contains a ridiculous number of calories. Most dining establishments will go out of their way to advertise nutritional information if it is good; if no information is available, you can assume it is bad.

Don't forget to keep track of everything you drink, even if the beverage has zero calories, like water or diet soda. You can work beer, wine, and liquor into your daily diet, but keep in mind that like sugary sodas they represent empty calories. Coffee and tea typically don't add calories if you drink yours without sugar or milk.

Deal with the short-term inconveniences of recording nutritional values now, and you will enjoy the benefits for a lifetime. Here are examples of a sample diet log for someone consuming 1,200, 1,700, and 2,100 calories per day:

DAILY FITNESS TRACKER

DATE: 5/22/07   DAY OF WEEK: TUESDAY

WATER INTAKE: ● ● ● ● ● ● ● ●

BREAKFAST	SERV	CAL	FAT	CARB	FIB	PRO	OTHER
Eggo waffle	1	120	5	16	0	3	
Strawberries	½ cup	23	0.3	5.2	1.7	0.5	
2% milk	1 cup	138	4.9	13.5	0	9.7	
LUNCH	SERV	CAL	FAT	CARB	FIB	PRO	
Chicken noodle soup	1 cup	75	2.4	9.3	0.7	4	
Saltine crackers	5	100	5	20.5	0.5	2.5	
Apple	1	81	0.5	21.1	3.7	0.3	
DINNER	SERV	CAL	FAT	CARB	FIB	PRO	
Pork loin	3 oz	199	11.4	0	0	22.3	
Baked potato	1	220	0.2	51	4.8	4.7	
Green beans	½ cup	22	0.2	4.9	2	1.2	
SNACK	SERV	CAL	FAT	CARB	FIB	PRO	
Air-popped popcorn	3 cups	93	0.9	18.6	3.6	3	
Peach	1	37	0.1	9.7	1.7	0.6	
Vanilla ice cream	½ cup	144	7.9	16.9	0.5	2.5	
DAILY TOTALS		CAL	FAT	CARB	FIB	PRO	OTHER
		1,252	38.8	186.7	19.2	54.3	

EXERCISE	DURATION	INTENSITY	CALORIES BURNED
Treadmill	60 min	Speed 3.5; incline 6	630

VITAMINS / QTY	SUPPLEMENTS / QTY	MEDICATIONS / QTY

DAILY JOURNAL

TODAY I FEEL:

DAILY FITNESS TRACKER

DATE: 5/22/07   DAY OF WEEK: TUESDAY

WATER INTAKE: ● ● ● ● ● ● ● ●

BREAKFAST	SERV	CAL	FAT	CARB	FIB	PRO	OTHER
Banana	1	105	0.6	26.7	2.7	1.2	
Bagel (plain)	1	150	1	34	1	9	
Peanut butter	2 tbsp	188	16	6.6	1.9	7.9	

LUNCH	SERV	CAL	FAT	CARB	FIB	PRO	
Wheat bread	2 slices	140	2	24	2.8	6	
Mayonnaise	1 tbsp	100	11	0	0	0	
Bologna (beef)	1 slice	88	8	0.6	0	3.3	
Cantaloupe	1 cup	58	0.4	13.4	1.2	1.4	

DINNER	SERV	CAL	FAT	CARB	FIB	PRO	
Chicken (light meat)	4 oz	196	5.1	0	0	35.1	
Broccoli	1 cup	24	0.4	4.6	2.6	2.6	
Pasta	1 cup cooked	197	0.9	39.7	2.4	6.7	
Butter	2 tbsp	200	22.8	0	0	0.2	

SNACK	SERV	CAL	FAT	CARB	FIB	PRO	
Chocolate chip cookie	1	130	6.9	16.7	0.9	0.9	
Cottage cheese	½ cup	100	2	4	0	0	
Carrot	1	31	0.1	7.3	2.2	0.7	

DAILY TOTALS		CAL	FAT	CARB	FIB	PRO	OTHER
		1,708	77.2	177.6	17.7	89	

EXERCISE	DURATION	INTENSITY	CALORIES BURNED
Tread-climber	60 min	3.0	938

VITAMINS / QTY	SUPPLEMENTS / QTY	MEDICATIONS / QTY

DAILY JOURNAL

TODAY I FEEL:

DAILY FITNESS TRACKER

DATE: 5/22/07 DAY OF WEEK: TUESDAY

WATER INTAKE: ● ● ● ● ● ● ● ●

BREAKFAST	SERV	CAL	FAT	CARB	FIB	PRO	OTHER
Orange juice	6 oz	80	0	20	0.1	0	
Cornflakes	2 oz	200	0	48	2	4	
2% milk	1 cup	138	4.9	13.5	0	9.7	
Blueberries	½ cup	41	0.3	10.2	2	0.5	

LUNCH	SERV	CAL	FAT	CARB	FIB	PRO	
Chili	1 cup	287	14	30.5	11	14.5	
Cheddar cheese	1 oz	110	9	1	0	7	
Saltine crackers	10	200	10	41	1	5	
Lettuce	2 cups	20	0.4	4	2	1.6	
Ranch dressing	2 tbsp	50	0	0	0	0	

DINNER	SERV	CAL	FAT	CARB	FIB	PRO	
Hamburger (80% lean)	4 oz	308	20.9	0	0	28	
Baked beans	½ cup	170	1	21	7	6	
Corn	½ cup	80	1	17	2	2	

SNACK	SERV	CAL	FAT	CARB	FIB	PRO	
Potato chips	15	160	10	14	1	2	
Brownie	1	220	13	27	1	1	
Watermelon	1 cup	50	0.6	11.4	0.8	1	

DAILY TOTALS		CAL	FAT	CARB	FIB	PRO	OTHER
		2,114	85.1	258.6	29.9	82.3	

EXERCISE	DURATION	INTENSITY	CALORIES BURNED
Bike	45 min	7	267
Stair-climber	15 min	4	137

VITAMINS / QTY	SUPPLEMENTS / QTY	MEDICATIONS / QTY

DAILY JOURNAL

TODAY I FEEL:

Keeping track of your food is really that easy, and the more you do it, the easier it becomes. You'll find that you eat many of the same foods throughout the week, so after a few days you won't have to look up the nutritional values for many of the items—the information you need will already be recorded in your diet log. What you learn about calorie counts will help you to control your portion sizes so that you can continue to eat the foods you like. If you eat healthy while you are losing weight, then these changes will be second nature when it comes time to maintain your loss.

DECODING LABELS

Read food labels very carefully and pay particular attention to two pitfalls: manufacturer advertising and portion sizes.

First, the name of the food and the advertising on the packaging can be totally misleading. I love Sun Chips and Wheat Thins, but Sun Chips do not come from the sun, and Wheat Thins are not made from pure wheat with nothing added. Brand names are designed to tempt you and often suggest that you are eating something healthy, even when you aren't. Some products advertise on the front of the bag: "Made with natural fruit flavors" and "Great multigrain *taste*." Flavor! Taste! Who cares? The ingredients matter more than the taste. What's in it? You need to read the food label yourself and decide if this is something you want to eat. Don't let a food company's marketing department make your food choices for you.

Second, pay close attention to the serving size listed on the food label. A package that looks like it contains a single serving often holds several. And if you're not careful, you'll wind up doubling the number of calories you intended to consume.

For example, Country Time Lemonade is sold in a box of six in-dividually wrapped drink packets. These packets are convenient: if you want some delicious lemonade but are in a hurry, you simply open the packet, pour the entire contents into a 16-ounce water bottle, and shake. The nutrition label says a single serving contains 35 calories, but, if you look closely, a single serving equals half of the little packet. So, if you drink the whole 16 ounces—which is easy to do and understandable since the packets aren't resealable—you've consumed 70 calories, not 35.

That bottle of juice? Probably has two servings, not one.

That small package of cookies? Could be three servings in there.

That "healthy" granola bar? Double-check that label.

Just because something looks small enough to be a single serv-ing doesn't mean it is one. Pay close attention to the serving size listed on each label, and record the accurate number of calories in your diet log.

MEASURING AND WEIGHING FOOD

You often have to weigh or measure your food to eat the proper serving size. Buy an inexpensive (about $10) scale in a health food store. An expensive scale with a digital screen and memory features is not a requirement. Just like a toaster or a blender, your scale will take its place on your kitchen counter. You can purchase a set of measuring cups at your supermarket or a kitchen-supply store.

Measuring and weighing food is important for two reasons. First, it eliminates guessing and estimating, which is diet suicide. When you measure and weigh your food, you know that the num-bers you record in your diet log are accurate, and it is easy to consis-tently lose weight. Second, by the time you reach your goal weight, you will have measured so many different foods so many times that it will be easy for you to look at a piece of turkey and say, "That is 3 ounces." If you don't measure and weigh food while you are losing pounds, you won't have the skill when it is time to maintain your weight.

Don't let the idea of measuring and weighing food frighten or discourage you; you'll get the hang of it. I used to cook pasta by filling the pan—and then filling my plate. When I started keeping track of my food, it was very strange to take a handful of pasta noodles, set them on a scale, and add or remove noodles until I had the amount of ounces I could eat that day. Now it's just part of my routine. The first couple of days will be difficult for you, but like everything else, it will become a habit soon enough.

COMPLICATED MEALS

How do you track complicated dishes that contain numerous ingredients, like my mom's famous lasagna? Sometime during our family's first month on the F.A.S.T. diet, my mother decided that she was going to make her famous lasagna for everyone. She figured out that she could make one pan, add up all of the nutrition numbers for the ingredients, and then divide the pan into equal servings. So she got to work. She bought three boxes of noodles and totaled the calories: 2,400. Then she added up the total for four bags of cheese: 1,890. Finally, the meat and sauce totaled 900 calories. The finished dish had 5,190 calories, 160 grams of fat, 518 grams of carbs, 96 grams of fiber, and 178 grams of protein. She cut the pan into ten equal pieces and, voilà, everyone (except me, because I don't like lasagna) had one piece of Mom's famous lasagna and recorded in their logs: 519 CAL, 12 FAT, 51.8 CARB, 9.6 FIB, and 17.8 PRO.

If you make dishes that require mixing several foods, the secret is to measure the first time. Write those numbers in a notebook or your diet log for future reference. After the first couple of weeks, tracking your food is easy because all your favorites now have nutritional values attached to them. To make it even easier for us, my mom made cards for each dish that listed the nutritional values. She copied them so that we could take a card home and insert the numbers in our logs. The cards looked like this:

Lasagna

Calories per serving	519
Fat	12
Carbs	51.8
Protein	17.8
Fiber	9.6

Enchiladas

Calories per enchilada	198
Fat	5
Carbs	27
Protein	11
Fiber	7

Taco Tot Casserole

Calories per serving	320
Fat	15
Carbs	29
Protein	12
Fiber	4

WHAT ABOUT GOING TO RESTAURANTS

I don't eat out very often, but many people do. The F.A.S.T. diet rule applies to eating out: *If you can't find the complete nutritional information for a food, then you can't eat it.* However, with a little planning you should be able to enjoy eating out. Just remember: you're the customer—don't let a menu dictate your health.

- Choose a diet-friendly restaurant that serves salads, vegetables, and baked or broiled entrées.
- Review the menu in advance and plan what you will order. Some restaurants even include nutritional information on their websites, so be sure to check.
- Don't be shy about asking for your meal to be prepared the way you want it. Order the chicken broiled, not fried. Ask for sauces and butter on the side. Skip high-calorie foods like potatoes and order steamed vegetables instead. Choose fruit for dessert instead of ice cream.
- Skip the beer or wine and have a nice big glass of ice water.

Sometimes it's not easy to make healthy choices or to plan ahead. In a pinch you can always eat a salad, which I hate, but it is much better than disregarding your diet.

The best advice for restaurant dining that I can give you is: *choose food that makes sense for your diet.* In the weight-loss phase of the F.A.S.T. diet, you must not make exceptions. When you get to the maintenance phase, you will be able to enjoy these exception foods from time to time.

Here's what you've learned so far about using the F.A.S.T. diet to lose weight and get healthy:

Three Days Before the First Weigh-in

- Don't change your eating habits but keep track of what you eat and drink in your diet log.
- Note any vitamins, supplements, or medications you are taking in your diet log.
- Don't eat a food unless you can find the complete nutritional information for it.

These steps will give you an accurate picture of your eating habits before you begin the F.A.S.T. diet *and* give you practice reading food labels.

Chapter 6

THE DIET: HOW WE ATE

I am going to solve a huge mystery for you right now. By the time you are finished reading this chapter, you are going to understand how to eat in order to lose weight. This information helped my family and one hundred volunteers in Omaha succeed. I am not a nutritionist or a doctor, and I encourage you to see one if you have questions or concerns about the F.A.S.T. diet. Talk to a professional before adjusting your diet if you have special needs that make you different from the average Joe.

To create the program we followed, I used information on diet and nutrition found on the Harvard School of Public Health website (hsph.harvard.edu) and at nutrition.gov. I also spoke to doctors and fitness professionals and consulted the sources listed at the back of the book (see Resources).

The F.A.S.T. program is very simple: calculate the minimum number of calories you need to function for one day and eat fewer calories than this by eating foods that you like. By keeping track of everything you eat to stay within your calorie limits, you'll learn the secret of moderation and how different foods affect your body. On the F.A.S.T. program you'll be able to eat a Snickers bar or a piece of cheesecake when you really want to or need to. (Yes, I said *need*. Don't we all need a Snickers bar every now and then?)

We live in a world where we have to make choices about food all the time. People often confuse what choices they actually have to make with the ones they need to make to get healthy. A person just starting a diet often thinks, Well, now that I am dieting, I guess that means no more ice cream. What, are you kidding? Who can diet successfully without ice cream? Not me! You will never succeed on a diet if you deprive yourself of the things you want to eat, even if they're junk food. This is the first rule our family made—*eat anything you want*. Just fit that item into the number of calories you have to work with that day.

I love Reese's peanut butter cups. They really are my all-time favorite food, even though they're not healthy in any way, shape, or form. I eat them all the time, and I ate them while I was dieting; in fact, I would have failed without them. When I started the F.A.S.T. diet, I was eating about 1,400 calories per day. A Reese's peanut butter cup is about 200 calories, so whenever I ate one, I did the math and subtracted 200 calories from my daily total, leaving 1,200 to eat. Sounds simple, right?

Have you ever been to The Cheesecake Factory? I love that place. Unfortunately, one piece of cheesecake equals about half the calories a person needs for an entire day. But that is a sacrifice I am sometimes willing to make. I think you should also make the sacrifice for your favorite foods. But don't indulge recklessly; work it into your plan in a way that doesn't undermine you. Eat your cheesecake, and if that means you're left with only 800 calories for the day, be careful to moderate your intake and only eat another 800 calories, no more. You *can* eat junk food and still be healthy: just be smart and work it into your daily plan instead of simply adding it on top of everything else.

I also love cheeseburgers. The place I go to serves these huge burgers that are 1,100 calories. Do I eat one and waste nearly all of my calories on one meal? I sure do, sometimes. If that is what I really want, I will eat it and then spread my remaining calories over the rest of the day. Should you do this every day? No. But could you do it once a week or once a month and be okay? Sure. Most people don't actually do this very often, though, because they prefer to spread calories throughout the day so they don't feel hungry. But it is nice to know you can indulge yourself once in a while.

Often when I explain this to people they say, "If I do that, I will be hungry all day. I can't do that." I understand this argument very well, but let me give you some perspective on what you are saying. Diet is as much of a physical game as it is a mental game; when you have thoughts like this, the mental game is taking advantage of you. If you're reading this book, you probably eat for a whole bunch of reasons that do not include physical hunger: boredom, stress, exhaustion, fear, nervousness, and love. If you only ate when you were hungry, then you wouldn't be overweight and you certainly would not be reading a diet book. See my point? *You are not hungry.* Your problem is not hunger; rather, you are eating too many unhealthy foods for all the wrong reasons—and your body is storing fat reserves. Children in the Sudan are hungry! You're probably just bored, saw a commercial about new white chocolate M&M's, and would like something to eat.

You may say, "Maybe you're not hungry, Tony, but I weigh 450 pounds and I need more food to survive." I agree you are big, Mr. 450, but let me say it again, "You are not hungry." Yes, you need nourishment, but eating is what a lot of us do to entertain ourselves when we are bored.

So, even though my family's first rule is to eat anything you want, *that does not mean you can eat as much of it as you want.*

THE F.A.S.T. DIET PLAN

Once you calculate how many calories you need in a day, then losing weight is a simple matter of eating less than that. You determine the number of calories you should eat each day using the Basal Metabolic Rate (BMR) formula.

The BMR is used by professional nutritionists to estimate how many calories you need to function for one day. It takes into account your height, age, and weight. Here is the formula for men and women:

$$Men: [66 + (6.3 \times current\ weight)$$
$$+ (12.9 \times height\ in\ inches)] - (6.8 \times age)$$
$$Women: [655 + (4.3 \times current\ weight)$$
$$+ (4.7 \times height\ in\ inches)] - (4.7 \times age)$$

So instead of eating only "perfect" foods, whole-grain this and tofu that, my family ate (and still eats) what we wanted to eat but stayed below the number of calories we calculated using the BMR formula. Many diets tell you that you have to eat only certain foods or the foods that they provide for you—I think this is crazy. In the real world, when you go to a party with friends, it's not likely they'll be serving a "Johnny Diets" low-cal dessert. Instead, they offer you a piece of rich chocolate cake. My teammates eat a small piece of that cake and then work the calories into their daily totals.

How far below your BMR number should you go to lose weight? Is lower better? Let's say you are a fifty-year-old woman who is five feet six and weighs 250 pounds. Your BMR number is 1,805 calories per day. If you eat less than that, in theory you will lose weight. Now for the magic number . . . 500 calories. Our goal was always to be 500 calories below our BMR number. Why? One pound equals 3,500 calories. There are seven days in a week, and if you are 500 calories below your BMR number, then you will burn exactly a pound per week. My doctor recommends never going below 1,000 calories if you are a woman or 1,200 if you are a man without permission from your own doctor.

These limits are very restrictive, but you should not violate them unless your doctor says to. If an older woman with a BMR of 1,250 calories were to lower her number by 500, then she would be well below the doctor-recommended minimum of 1,000 calories. This cannot happen. The lowest this woman could go to would be 1,000 calories. That leaves a deficit of 250 calories, or a half pound per week. If this woman wants to lose more than a half pound per week, the answer is exercise. If she burns 250 calories a day in exercise, she reaches her 500-calorie-per-day deficit. Watch the pounds fly off! Some big men will have very high BMR numbers. I don't recommend that they go below 500 calories (750 max) of their BMR; it is too easy to get hungry and then it is more tempting to cheat.

Have you figured out your number? Great!

Once you have calculated your number, then use the chart on page 102 to guide your daily intake of carbs, fats, and proteins. Again, I am not a nutritionist, but here is the daily breakdown that worked for me and my family. We created this chart from the information provided at nutrition.gov. Our goal was for approximately 60 percent of our calories to come from carbohydrates so that our bodies would have plenty of fuel. Protein was 20 percent or more of our calories but never more than 40 percent to give our bodies the building blocks they needed to build and repair muscle. Fats accounted for about 20 percent of our calorie intake.

Calories per day	Carb (grams)	Protein (grams)	Fat (grams)
1,250	188	63	42
1,300	195	65	43
1,350	203	68	45
1,400	210	70	47
1,450	218	73	48
1,500	225	75	50
1,550	233	78	52
1,600	240	80	53

If you stay within these levels, you'll lose 1 to 2 pounds per week. Let's review what you'll be tracking.

CARBOHYDRATES

All the bad information you read about carbohydrates drives me mad. I can hardly believe that anyone would promote a low-carb diet. Carbohydrates are the main source of energy for our bodies. I suppose that people are so starved for the ultimate answer to the diet-and-obesity crisis that you can tell them just about anything, and if it seems like a quick fix, they will believe it. The truth is, you need carbs; in fact, many of the foods that are good for you contain carbs. I want you to imagine for a second how long you could run your car without fuel. Sure, it would run on fumes for a while, but pretty soon it would stop. You need fuel to run your car, and you need carbs to run your body.

Rather than pay too much attention to how many carbs we ate, my family carefully watched the kinds of carbs we ate. Carbs are categorized as complex or simple, and it is very important for you to understand the difference between the two, because once you do, you'll have solved almost effortlessly dieting's biggest problem—hunger.

Simple carbohydrates are simple because they break down very quickly into sugar, which is then used for energy. Sometimes this whole process takes only thirty minutes. The sugar in soda is a simple carb: all the energy from the soda is transported into the bloodstream very quickly to use for fuel. The process allows too much energy to be released into your body too quickly; this fast "sugar high" is followed by an equally fast low. Imagine putting gas into your car's tank with a fire hose; sure, you'd get some fuel in the tank, but it would be too much too quick. Here is a list of foods that contain simple carbohydrates:

Table sugar
Corn syrup (high-fructose corn syrup)
Fruit juice
Candy
Soda pop
All baked goods made with white flour
Pasta made with white flour
Most packaged cereals

Complex carbohydrates are much more difficult to break down into sugar in your stomach. These foods can take as long as four hours to break down into the sugar that gets released into your bloodstream. Instead of getting a huge sugar rush, you are less likely to get hungry and therefore more likely to be successful dieting. No big high and no big low means a continuous, consistent flow of energy. If the majority of the carbs you eat are complex carbs, you have nothing to worry about: they are great for you.

Here is a list of foods that contain complex carbohydrates:

Apples	Grapefruit	Radishes
Apricots	Kidney beans	Skim milk
Artichokes	Lentils	Soybeans
Asparagus	Lettuce	Soy milk
Broccoli	Multigrain	Spinach
Brown rice	bread	Split peas
Brussels sprouts	Navy beans	Strawberries
Buckwheat	Oat bran bread	Tomatoes
and buckwheat	and cereal	Turnip greens
bread	Oatmeal	Watercress
Cabbage	Okra	Whole barley
Carrots	Onions	Whole-meal
Cauliflower	Oranges	spelt bread
Celery	Pears	Wild rice
Cucumbers	Pinto beans	Yams
Dill pickles	Plums	Yogurt
Eggplant	Potatoes	(low fat)
Garbanzo beans	Prunes	Zucchini

Don't try to run your car without gas and definitely don't try to run your body without fuel. *Lowering carbohydrate intake by itself will not cause you to lose weight.* If you are eating all protein or all fat or all anything and your calories are above the amount you need per day, you will gain weight whether you are eating carbs or eating dirt; it makes little difference. Instead of depriving your body of anything, the secret is to find the right balance. And that balance should always include carbs.

PROTEINS

Proteins are the building blocks of your body, and on the F.A.S.T. diet we paid very close attention to our protein intake. Since we were exercising every single day, we often had sore muscles. Yes, you will be sore, too! Protein is what your body uses to heal these sore muscles. Excess protein can also be used as an energy source, but not as efficiently as carbs, so our goal was always to stay above the protein number we listed on the chart on page 102 and below whatever that number would be doubled.

The secret to getting the right proteins is actually very simple unless you are a vegetarian, in which case it is a bit more complicated. Variety is the key; eat a lot of different types of high-protein foods. The ones that give you the most bang for your buck are animal proteins found in meat, milk, and cheese, which are called whole, or complete, proteins. To make it very simple, imagine a puzzle with ten pieces. Some proteins don't come with all the pieces; they may have only five or six, so you need to eat something else to complement that meal to make a full puzzle. This is why vegetarians will eat beans and rice together, because the two of them combined make a complete protein: one has six pieces of the puzzle and the other has the missing four, and together they make a whole protein.

Animal proteins don't have this problem. Instead, they have all ten pieces from the start, so if you can eat them and like them, they are an excellent choice, especially lean meats like fish and chicken. Soy contains protein equal to that of animal sources. Vegetarians should do more research to find the right protein combinations: consult books like *The New Becoming Vegetarian* by Melinda Vesanto and Brenda Davis and other sources listed in "Resources" (page 247). The person who eats an average, varied diet that includes some meat will get plenty of the right proteins.

Protein was always the last thing we would ask each other about at our daily check-ins, but you will need to get enough in your diet so your body can repair those sore muscles. Cheeseburger, anyone?

FATS

I love fat. Fat makes me happy because it comes in all the foods I love, like Reese's peanut butter cups. Cheesecake is also a high-fat food, although there are some good low-fat or nonfat substitutes. We all eat these foods, and I hope you won't give up your favorite fatty foods: just don't eat them like a bear that just finished hibernating and accidentally ran into a sleeping antelope five minutes after he stepped out of his cave in spring; eat them with moderation—especially the ones that have the bad fats.

How do you tell the difference between bad fats and good fats?

Bad Fats

Trans fats are the really bad ones. According to U.S. nutritional guidelines, there is no safe limit of trans fats that you can consume daily—not even 1 gram. Trans fats must be listed on food nutrition labels, so it's easy for you to know how much you're consuming. Do I eat them anyway? Yes. Do I understand that they are poison to my body? Yes. Do I understand that they raise my bad cholesterol and lower my good? Yes, so I use moderation: if a food I really like has trans fats, I may eat it only once or twice a month. I never give it up entirely, but I am aware of how much I am putting in my body. Because of the danger of trans fats, they are starting to get some serious attention; in fact, the New York City Board of Health unanimously voted to ban all artificial trans fats in city restaurants by July 2008. Can you believe that? New York made it a law that restaurants could not serve trans fats. Pretty soon people in New York will be boot-legging trans fats: a guy will lean over to his waiter, slip him $20, and say, "Hey, Jimmy, how about getting me a piece of that . . . special cheesecake in the back." Who knows? Seriously, though, trans fats are very bad for you.

Saturated fats are not nearly as bad for you as trans fats, but you definitely want to limit your intake of them. U.S. nutritional guide-lines recommend that you stay below 20 grams per day, which is more than you think, especially if most of your diet consists of high-fiber foods that rarely contain much saturated fat. Saturated fats raise your bad cholesterol, but they raise your good cholesterol, too. When a food I love is high in saturated fats, sometimes I will eat it every day of the week as long as I am staying below my daily recom-mended intake of 20 grams.

Good Fats

Good fats are called *polyunsaturated* and *monounsaturated fats*. Peo-ple often don't understand the concept of "good" fats. How can a fat be good when there has been so much bad press about fats over the past few years? After all, everything we eat says low fat or no fat. Let me clarify: vitamins are good; wheat and grain are good; fruits and vegetables are good; and, in the same way, poly- and monounsatu-rated fats are good. There is only one thing wrong with them: they are high in calories and harder than carbs to fit into your daily caloric intake. The reason they are so good for you is because they do exactly the opposite of what trans fats do: *raise your good choles-terol and lower your bad cholesterol*. In fact, they are so good for your overall health that they should actually be called "great fats."

Here is a list of foods that contain good fats (polyunsaturated and monounsaturated):

Almonds
Avocados
Canola oil
Cashews
Fish
Flaxseeds
Mayonnaise
Olive oil
Olives
Peanut butter
Peanut oil
Peanuts
Pecans
Salad dressing
Sesame oil
Shellfish
Sunflower seeds

My family's goal was to always stay below the fat grams listed in the chart on page 102. It is okay to exceed that number as long as you are not eating a lot of bad fat and not exceeding your daily calorie limits.

FIBER

Fiber is a carbohydrate that your body uses as a cleanser—it's the maid that cleans the house that is your body. Fiber attaches itself to the trash in your body and then carries the waste out. The best thing about fiber is that your body can't digest all of it so you feel full longer. Fiber is essential to success on the F.A.S.T. plan. On food labels you will see that some foods are loaded with fiber, but when food manufacturers do the math for the calories, they assign no calories to this fiber. In theory, a food could have 0 grams of fat, 19 grams of fiber, and 0 grams of protein and be listed as having 0 calories. Because of this, fiber is almost like a free food. (Now, if chocolate cake only had more fiber...)

According to the experts, you need a minimum of 25 grams of fiber per day and should stay below 40 grams. When my family first started the F.A.S.T. diet, it seemed like it was going to be hard to get so much fiber, so one of the things we did as a team was to find high-fiber foods we actually enjoyed. It became like a treasure hunt to us.

Here is a list of foods that are high in fiber. You can research more high-fiber foods on websites like http://www.mayoclinic .com/health/high-fiber-foods/NU00582 and http://www.hsph .harvard.edu/nutritionsource/fiber.html.

Fruits	Serving Size	Total Fiber (grams)
Pear	1 medium	5.1
Figs (dried)	2 medium	3.7
Blueberries	1 cup	3.5
Apple (with skin)	1 medium	3.3
Strawberries	1 cup	3.3
Peaches (dried)	3 halves	3.2
Orange	1 medium	3.1
Apricots (dried)	10 halves	2.6
Raisins	1.5-oz box	1.6
Grains, Cereal, and Pasta		
Spaghetti (whole wheat)	1 cup	6.3
Bran flakes	¾ cup	5.1
Oatmeal	1 cup	4.0
Bread (rye)	1 slice	1.9
Bread (whole wheat)	1 slice	1.9
Bread (mixed grain)	1 slice	1.7
Bread (cracked wheat)	1 slice	1.4

Legumes and Nuts	Serving Size	Total Fiber (grams)
Lentils	1 cup	15.6
Black beans	1 cup	15.0
Lima beans	1 cup	13.2
Baked beans (canned)	1 cup	10.4
Almonds	24 nuts	3.3
Pistachios	47 nuts	2.9
Peanuts	28 nuts	2.3
Cashews	18 nuts	0.9
Vegetables		
Peas	1 cup	8.8
Artichoke (cooked)	1 medium	6.5
Brussels sprouts	1 cup	6.4
Turnip greens (boiled)	1 cup	5.0
Potato (baked)	1 medium	4.4
Corn	1 cup	4.2
Popcorn (air popped)	3 cups	3.6
Tomato paste	1/4 cup	3.0
Carrot	1 medium	2.0

Reading labels allowed us to create our own lists of prepared and packaged high-fiber foods that we could buy at our local supermarket. The differences in fiber for two very similar foods can be drastic. For example, some fajita shells have 1 gram of fiber per serving and some have 26 grams. Both taste great. By carefully reading labels you can choose healthier versions of foods you already like. This will make it easier for you to get and remain healthy. On most food labels fiber is listed under "carbohydrates" as "dietary fiber."

Occasionally you will buy something that is very high in fiber, try it, and hate it. No big deal—just don't buy it again. Soon you will compile a whole list of delicious foods that are loaded with fiber. You must like the foods you are eating because that is the only way you will ever be able to lose weight consistently and then maintain your goal weight when you reach it. It is nearly impossible to succeed if you don't like the food, so keep looking until you find high-fiber foods you enjoy.

You will notice a change within days once you start increasing your fiber. Your energy levels will rise drastically because your body is no longer storing extra waste and trash in your body. The fiber flushes it out. When you add fiber to your diet, you will immediately see a change in your stool. This softer, easier-to-pass waste will help eliminate future health problems such as hemorrhoids.

Most people don't get enough fiber. Many people on the F.A.S.T. diet lose more than 10 pounds in the first week because of the flushing-out process. This is not a sustainable weight loss, and if you do lose that much, don't expect it to continue. The goal each week is to lose anywhere from 1 to 2.5 pounds.

Eat lots of fiber!

WATER

Undoubtedly someone has told you that you should drink eight glasses of water a day. But do you know why?

Because water is critical to your overall health, and most of us do not get enough of it. Sure, we get enough water just to get by, but not enough to function at our highest level, or even close to it. Water plays the role in your body that oil does in the engine of your car. According to the experts, you should drink at least eight 8-ounce glasses a day. However, I believe that if you are really working out hard, as you should be, then ten glasses are better. Actually, this was the minimum intake for our family. We got our best results when we drank much of the water with meals. Sixteen ounces with each meal really helped our bodies to digest, distribute, and process the food into energy. Plus, when you drink more water, your stomach is full, and you tend not to be hungry, which means less desire to overeat.

In an attempt to beat the system, some people will substitute iced tea, diet soda, or juice for water, but these fluids are not as good. Your body needs plain water. Some people think that bottled water tastes better, and if you can afford it and prefer it, that's fine. But plain old tap water, as long as it is safe, is all your body really needs. If the only way you can get the water into your system is to drink flavored waters, then that is certainly better than no water at all.

If you drink lots of water, you will increase your energy and physical vibrancy. You will feel more alert and sleep better at night. (Unless, of course, you drink water right before you go to bed; then you won't sleep at all.) You will notice that your skin is clearer and feels softer. My parents had rough patches on their elbows and feet that had been there for years. As they increased their water intake, these skin conditions cleared up. If you come down with the flu or a cold, take your doctor's advice and drown that cold in water; your body will respond and recover quickly.

On the F.A.S.T. plan, the first question a teammate asks during the daily check-in is "How much water did you have?" If the answer is not eight or more glasses, the person is tied to a pole and gets one lash for each glass missed. Seriously, water intake is a priority in the F.A.S.T. diet because it really is crucial to our success.

By the way, did I mention that water is calorie free? Drink away!

MAKE BETTER FOOD CHOICES

As long as you stay within the parameters outlined above, you can eat anything you want on the F.A.S.T. diet. After just a couple of days, people start to lose weight and feel so good that they *want* to eat better foods. Here are some suggestions to help you make healthier food choices:

- Retrain your taste buds slowly. I have learned that when we make easy food choices we make bad food choices. Unfortunately, whole grains and fruits do not grow in vending machines or soda cans. To make matters worse, we think that a lot of the bad stuff we eat tastes better than the good stuff; however, this is not true. The true issue is not one of taste but of training. You can get used to just about anything, and the taste of food is no different: once you start adding healthy foods to your diet and liking them, you will crave them over the junk you used to eat.

  For example, don't switch from whole milk to skim milk cold turkey; instead, ease into it slowly. When you want a glass of milk, fill it three-quarters with whole milk and a quarter with skim. It won't make enough of a difference for you to notice, and the milk will taste just fine. After one week, make the milk a fifty-fifty blend, and your taste buds will adjust again. After another week, fill the glass with 75 percent skim milk and 25 percent whole milk; your taste buds will adjust again. Finally, drink 100 percent skim milk: it will taste good and whole milk will taste thick and undrinkable.

  You can apply this same process to many of your foods. I used to love white rice. I could eat bowls and bowls of it. Pasta, too. But I slowly integrated brown rice and whole-wheat pasta into my diet, and now they taste great to me. The benefits are amazing. Brown rice and whole-wheat pasta are complex carbohydrates and break down into sugar much slower than their white counterparts. So instead of getting a sugar rush and being hungry again in twenty minutes, I have a continuous supply of energy for hours. When I eat white rice now, I almost feel sick.

If you are a cheese lover, don't despair. Low-calorie, low-fat cheese tastes great. Try just a few servings, and you will prefer it to thick, bulky regular cheese. Don't make all of these changes at once; look for better choices to gradually replace the foods you are already eating. Often you'll find alternatives that taste as good or better than what you are eating. Your body will adjust as you get healthier and soon you will want only the foods that are best for you.

■ Don't rely on willpower. That is why you are reading this book in the first place; you don't have any and neither did we. Sometimes making the healthy food choice is a matter of planning for that moment when you know you will struggle. For example, grocery shopping while you are hungry is insane. Everything that winds up in your cart will be chocolate or ice cream or chocolate ice cream. Instead, eat first, then shop. Another tip is to remove temptations from your house. I never think about or want a Pepsi until I see one. I could go a year without having a can, but once it's in our house, I crave it. You probably could list a dozen foods like this: ice cream, chips, candy, and so on. Although you might be strong now, remember that you're just ten minutes away from dipping chocolate bars in peanut butter and washing them down with big spoonfuls of rocky road. Sometimes the trick to making the healthy choice is making it before the moment comes when you can't control yourself. Get those temptations out of the house.

Cutting back on chocolate can be especially difficult. Men love chocolate, and women sometimes *need* chocolate. Once you start dieting, this *will not* change. So when your craving hits, make sure you have an alternative on hand that will give you your chocolate fix without a lot of empty calories. The best solutions we have found are low-calorie fudge bars with as few as 35 calories each and 3 grams of fiber—plus they taste great—and a low-calorie cupcake with creme filling (three total 100 calories and 5 grams of fiber). The cupcakes are very small, but if you need some chocolate, either of these will satisfy your craving without destroying your diet. I'm sure you'll find a lot of options at your grocery store—just read the labels carefully.

Remember

- Don't exceed the number of calories you should eat based on your BMR.
- Drink no less than eight glasses of water a day.
- Try very hard to eat between 25 and 40 grams of fiber per day.
- Try very hard to exceed your daily protein requirement but do not double it.
- Eat as much polyunsaturated and monounsaturated fat as you can fit into your daily calorie plan; limit saturated fat to 20 grams per day; avoid trans fats altogether if possible.
- Make carbs, preferably complex carbs, the centerpiece of your diet.

Once we had calculated our BMRs and our basic daily nutrition requirements, we were able to take control of what we ate. Our goals were to eat foods we liked, stay 500 calories below our BMR numbers, and learn how to be healthy for the rest of our lives. Exercise would become an integral part of that health strategy. So now let me share how our exercises plan worked. You might want to grab a towel for the next chapter—you're going to sweat.

Chapter 7

GREAT WORKOUTS: WINNING THE MENTAL GAME

There really is something strange about walking into a gym for the first time. It feels so uncomfortable, doesn't it? What is so ironic about that feeling is that the gym is the place you need to be most when you feel that way. It would be like feeling strange about going to the doctor when you are sick. If you are nervous about going for the first time, don't be. That is where you belong. Soon you will be walking around the gym like you own the place.

A long time ago I walked into a pizza place I used to frequent and the guy behind the counter said, "Hey, Tony, you want the regular?" I said, "Sure." He knew exactly what I wanted, my favorite pizza—green peppers and cheese. I thought this was so cool. I walk in and he knows me by my first name; I'm famous. Then I realized something bad. That night when I got home, I said to my wife, "Sweetheart, I just learned a lesson about life, and a quick way to determine how you are doing. Wherever they know your name by heart, that is an easy way to gauge the direction your life is going."

For example, remember on the show *Cheers* when Norm walked in and everyone would say, "NORM!" When everyone at the bar knows your name, you're probably spending too much time there. It was the same for me at the pizza place, because as far as I can tell, pizza is not health food yet (but I am working on it). On the other hand, if you walk into your stockbroker's office and he knows your name, that's a good sign. Well, the same goes for the gym: if there is anywhere you want to be popular, this is it.

When our family first went to the gym, everyone was nervous, and most of us had only two-week passes. We went late at night so there would be no crowds. We headed quickly to the treadmills; after all, we could all walk, so we figured that might be the place to start. What happened next was so much worse than I could have expected. Not only could no one run, but most of the group could barely walk for more than a minute or two without serious strain. The whole family was on level 1, and they looked like they were going to pass out after ten minutes. Everyone's feet hurt, backs were sore, and so on. If you can run from your front door to your car in the driveway, you are in ten times better shape than anyone in my family was that night. They were really hurting, and everyone wanted to quit.

After thirty minutes, they all got off the machines. My parents had to be helped off because they were so wobbly. Watching my dad walk was like watching a much older man struggle to his walker before he fell. I even suggested that they ask someone to drive them home afterward. It was that bad.

But it was also that good! We had all done it—thirty minutes each on the treadmill. For the next twenty minutes it was nothing but high fives and "Way to go's."

We learned an important lesson on that first day, one that is critical to your overall success in this program. Pay close attention to it:

You can accomplish any goal, if you work
toward it a little bit each day.

When people think about dieting and getting healthy, they lose sight of the here and now and focus only on the big picture: "You mean I have to work out *every day* for the rest of my life?" Most times I would advocate a big-picture view of the world, but when it comes to losing weight and getting fit, this is the wrong way to do it.

Although you might have to work out every day for the rest of your life . . . you don't have to do it all *today*. You only have to do *one* workout today, that's all. Concentrate only on today and deal with tomorrow when it comes.

Imagine how overwhelming raising a child would seem if you thought, You mean I have to raise her every day for the rest of my life, and then when she is finally out of the house, I still have to keep helping her through every little problem? Although it is a huge chore if we look at the entire picture, the fact is, we don't raise our children all in one day. We do a little bit today and a little bit tomorrow, but almost no day goes by when we don't do something to influence their lives. If your child is responsible, has good manners, and is hardworking, it is not because you worked real hard and were a great parent for one day. It is because you did a little bit each day over a lifetime. A little today and a little tomorrow. Your health is no different; it just takes an hour today and an hour tomorrow. You can't make up a missed workout from yesterday, so don't try. You can only affect today, so make it good.

When we break raising our children down into individual days and tasks, it becomes manageable. You need to handle your exercise and diet the same way.

And that is exactly what my family did. We exercised for thirty to sixty minutes each day. Instead of focusing on the level we exercised at, we paid attention to the calories burned. Each day's goal was to beat the previous day's calories burned. This forced us to improve ourselves and continue to work harder than we did the day before. We learned very quickly an important lesson about exercise: *consistency and constant improvement are the recipe for success when it comes to exercise (and actually in most things in life as well)*. The more days you exercise in a row without missing a session, the quicker your health will improve and the faster you will lose weight. Working out thirty days randomly in a year will have almost no impact on your health, but working out thirty days in a row will have a substantial impact. Second, don't try to fit exercise into your life. The sooner you realize that you must work your life around exercise, the sooner you will create the habits that will springboard you to amazing health.

When we started the F.A.S.T. program in November 2005, there was a lot of debate about what our exercise regimen should look like and how it could be tailored to each person so no one was overworked, which would likely cause injuries, and no one was underworked, which would likely mean no results. When creating this balance of working out hard but not too hard, my family had to face a huge problem: everyone was out of shape in a serious way and almost none of us had a clue what to do. It is really important that you understand what I mean when I say, *we were extremely out of shape.*

Both of my parents were more than 100 pounds overweight and had smoked and drank for at least twenty-five years. My sisters were all developing what they called Big Bertha butts, and none could run up a flight of stairs without getting winded. No one in my family went to the gym except for Jamie, who was going a couple of days a week but was still more than 100 pounds overweight. Jeremy smoked and was 80 pounds overweight, Julie was pregnant and 100 pounds overweight, and I had a torn Achilles. We were a mess. On top of all this, no one except me knew the difference between a dumbbell and a barbell. In fact, when it came to exercise, we were all dumbbells.

Here is the exercise plan that we finally decided on:

1. We would exercise every day, no exceptions.
2. We would do resistance training for two days out of the seven, which would include lifting free weights or using weight-lifting machines.
3. We would do cardio for thirty to sixty minutes each day for the other five days.

Although cardio is defined as any activity that raises your heart rate to a level where you're working but can still talk, we decided that the exercise would have to be on a machine that would track calories burned on a digital display, such as a treadmill, stair-climber, stationary bike, elliptical trainer, or rowing machine.

When I came up with the cardio plan, it complicated things a bit because it meant no walking or running except on a treadmill and no swimming. Things like gardening or mowing the lawn would also not count toward our daily exercise. Since then, we have made some changes that allow walking, running, and swimming to accomplish the same goal over a slightly longer time.

THE CARDIO PLAN

Cardio is a great way for you to burn calories and lose weight. And it provides a lot of other benefits:

- Strengthens your heart so that it doesn't have to work as hard to pump blood.
- Increases your lung capacity.

- Reduces the risk of heart attack, high cholesterol, high blood pressure, and diabetes.
- Boosts your confidence. Things that used to be heavy are suddenly light. A task that used to wear you down in an hour can be done all day and you feel great.
- Adds two hours to your life for every hour of cardio, according to the American Heart Association. Let that sink in and then tell me you don't have time to work out.

And, once you get going, you'll feel great.

When someone joins the F.A.S.T. program, he or she usually asks why the exercise has to be done on a machine. The reason is actually very simple and makes a lot of sense. If you are going to get healthy, you need to exercise regularly, but you also need to improve or increase your level of effort. This is very tricky for most people when they start the program because they are so out of shape. We solved the need to be able to track consistent improvement in our exercise by adopting *exercise rule #1:*

> *Always do better today than you did the last time,
> even if it is just a little bit.*

This rule forces you to measure what you are doing so that you can easily tell if you are working harder or slacking off. For example, let's say you are walking on a Nautilus 7000 treadmill at the gym. The first time you get on the treadmill you should take it very easy. Walk as slow or as fast as you like, at a level that is comfortable and at which you are not likely to hurt yourself. Once you have completed at least thirty minutes and no more than sixty minutes, stop and look at the calories you burned. Let's say it was 117. Great! Congratulate yourself; you have just completed a workout. Then go home and write the number in your diet log. Include the type of machine you used, how many minutes you worked out, and how many calories you burned. It is also useful to include any settings, so if you set the speed to 3.5 and the incline to 5.0, record this as well. As you start to break your own records, you'll be amazed that at six months down the road you are now working twice as hard and sweating half as much.

It really does not matter how many calories you burn at your first workout. What matters is what you do at your next workout. Tomorrow it's time to work out again. You have decided to use the Nautilus 7000 again, but how hard should you work out today? The answer is, "Harder than last time." You have improved even if you beat your last workout by only a single calorie. It makes no difference how much you improve, it just matters that you are improving. These tiny improvements add up quickly. My sixty-year-old father burned 124 calories at his first workout and slowly improved on it day by day; now he can burn almost 1,100 calories in an hour. My fifty-six-year-old mom can burn almost 850 calories in an hour; several of my sisters can run for at least an hour now.

Imagine that first block placed at the bottom of the Great Pyramid. It couldn't have looked like much, but without that first block, you never get to put the top one on. One piece, one workout, one day at a time will have a huge impact on your health and much faster than you think.

Finally, after a few weeks, you're up to 245 calories per workout. When you arrive at the gym today, someone else is using the Nautilus 7000. You were all excited to get on it and make a new personal record. You look around and see another machine called the Lifecycle 8500. So you get on that and start huffing and puffing; you give it your best effort for thirty minutes and look down at the calories burned. "Only 197? How can that be?" Suddenly you are confused because you worked so hard and burned fewer calories. Believe me, this will happen to you. When it does, remember exercise rule #1: *always do better today than you did the last time, even if it is just a little bit.*

I am sure you are thinking, But that is what I tried to do, and it didn't work because I burned fewer calories. Here is the trick: improvements must be measured on the same machine, because machines are very different. One treadmill will show you burning 300 calories and another only 150 calories with the same effort. So don't beat yourself up. Instead, make this day 1 on the new machine. Pat yourself on the back for completing another great workout, and the next time you are on the Lifecycle 8500, try to beat 197 calories.

Get it? Good! A few weeks later you are ready to try some of the harder machines. You have been feeling good and think you are finally up to the task. So you jump on the hardest machine in the gym: the Power Body 3500 cross-trainer. This machine works your arms, back, legs, and every other muscle you have hard. After really pushing yourself for thirty minutes you look down and see you have burned 429 calories. Wow, congratulations. Should you be excited? Yes, of course you should. But should you compare this number to your treadmill results? Absolutely not. Once again, you are looking for improvements on a machine-by-machine basis. So your new goal is to beat 429 calories burned the next time you are brave enough to step on the Power Body 3500. This is why my family works out on machines, because it is easy to measure exactly how wc are or aren't improving. If you go for a leisurely walk in the park, you'd rarely walk the same path, and there'd be no way to tell how hard you are working out. The amount of time you worked out is not nearly as important as the amount of effort and the rate of your improvement.

By now you are probably thinking that you don't want to work out on machines for the rest of your life: you like to walk and love to run. Maybe swimming gives you pleasure. There are hundreds of other workout options: an exercise DVD, Spinning classes, kickboxing, dance, and so on. Those are great choices to help you maintain, but while you are losing the weight, you really need a gauge not only to keep track of your progress but also to make you accountable, and machines do this. Although the other workouts may be great, there is no way to calculate your progress, so there is no accountability. At the end of a kickboxing workout, you could have really gone all out and had been covered in sweat or you could have totally slacked off. When you finish, all you know is that you're done. At the end of a machine workout, though, the digital display gives you a number. That number will tell you exactly if you are doing better or worse: if you burned only 250 calories today and 300 yesterday, then you know that you did not work as hard as you could have. Today there is no way you can talk yourself into thinking that you did better, because the numbers are right in front of you. And the numbers never lie! In kickboxing class, you can say things like "I know I didn't work that hard but at least I went." Pretty soon, you're coasting and can't figure out why you aren't losing weight.

But let's say that you are adamant about walking or running, or let's say you are what we affectionately call a Grand Fatty and walking is the only exercise you can do. That is fine, but to succeed you must also learn to track your exercise level so that you can slowly improve from day to day. Let's say today is day 1 on your walk and you have decided to walk for exactly thirty minutes. Perfect. Get a good stopwatch so you can know exactly when you are done. Before you begin walking, mark your starting point (your house, for example). As the thirty minutes is coming to a close, note where you are. Are you standing by the high school or are you standing by a fire hydrant? Write down the spot in your diet log. The next day, walk for exactly thirty minutes again, but try to walk farther than the spot where you stopped yesterday. Because you have a goal, you will soon find that you are walking much faster and improving each day, and that is the only thing we are trying to accomplish each day in exercise.

Never exercise superhard when you first start, or you'll hurt yourself and delay your progress. Take it slow; try to increase the level of your workouts by small increments. Remember, it has taken ten or more years for some people to gain all this extra weight— years of hardcore overeating. Think of all the times you had three cheeseburgers when you should have had only one. Think of all the times you stood at the McDonald's counter with a supersize Coke and French fries in your hand thinking, Hey, is there any way to *supersize* a supersize? Now you are finally going to reverse all that overindulgence. Most people are able to undo the damage in less than a year. That may seem like a long time, but it's much faster than how long it took to add those pounds.

If all you want to do is swim, and I can't convince you that the machines will give the best results, then you have to count laps and wear a waterproof stopwatch to track your time. If you do thirty laps in thirty minutes today you'll need to swim thirty-one laps in the same time tomorrow. You must always choose a time and beat your laps in the same interval. Pretty soon you will be swimming like a fish. Water aerobics are a terrible choice for most people because there is no way for you to track how hard you worked. Don't do them, unless you are so obese that this is your only choice. As soon as you lose some weight, start swimming or walking on the treadmill instead.

Your gym may have thirty machines of all shapes and sizes, and you need to master them all, but not today and not all at once. Don't be afraid to try new programs on the equipment. Ask the staff to help you. My family has learned the intricacies of each machine. When one of us gets on the stair-climber, for example, he or she

knows exactly which program burns the most calories in the short-
est time. The only way you will ever learn this yourself is by experi-
menting constantly. And you may be able to rule a machine that a
teammate can barely handle. I have trouble keeping up with my
sixty-year-old father, a former smoker and hard drinker, on the
treadmill. For some reason he is just great at it—we call him the Sul-
tan of the Treadmill. Variety will help you succeed. The machines
don't bite, so learn how they work and have fun.

RESISTANCE TRAINING

Lifting weights is the easiest exercise of all, but many people are
scared of it. Before I explain how your weight program will work, I
want to share with you my favorite weight-lifting story and biggest
pet peeve.

Before starting the F.A.S.T. program, I had spent a lot of money
on hundreds of personal training sessions with Ramsay Geha, a
friend of mine who looks like a grizzly bear. The time I spent with
Ramsay not only helped me get much stronger but also taught me
many lessons that I now pass on to other people.

Now for the funny part: Every time I take someone to the gym
to lift weights for the first time, he or she always says the same
thing: "I'm looking to tone a little here and there, but I don't want to
get *huge*. I don't want to look like one of those bodybuilders." I am
always stunned to hear this. Weight lifting and bodybuilding are serious sports; to build any muscle at all you have to work out at a
pro-athlete level. You really have to commit to a serious lifting regimen. Plus weight lifters eat nonstop, sometimes as much as 8,000
calories per day. As you can imagine, that doesn't fit well into the
F.A.S.T. plan.

Casual lifting cannot accidentally make you huge. It makes me laugh when people think that they will wake up one morning after a good workout, look in the mirror, and realize that they became huge overnight. "Oh, great, look what happened, I go to the gym one day and now I am huge." So don't worry, you won't get huge!

The level of weight lifting that we will be doing offers some amazing benefits, though. You will first notice a slight change in your strength and maybe in the size of your muscles, which always boosts your confidence. Resistance training strengthens bone and slows down bone loss. But what you will like the most is the pride and confidence that come with feeling stronger. Lifting weights really is fun; you will learn to love it.

Now, on to the workouts.

Everyone on the F.A.S.T. program does the same resistance training regimen: two days of lifting weights/resistance training each week. If you are new to weight lifting/resistance training, see page 128.

Day 1: Chest, Biceps, Triceps, Shoulders, and Back

To work each of these body parts, do three sets of ten repetitions with any weight that you can lift without straining. Track your results so that you can be accountable and try to do better next time. Let's say that today you chose to do the bench press, which is a chest exercise, and you did three sets of ten repetitions with 50 pounds; at your next session, try to do the same number of sets with 55 pounds, or do three sets of eleven repetitions with 50 pounds. Any improvement is the goal. After a couple of days of cardio it is time to do your second round of weight lifting.

Day 2: Quads, Hamstrings, Calves, and Abdominals

Do three sets of ten repetitions with any weight that you can lift without straining. Keep track of your results and try to beat your efforts next time.

Advice for the Novice

What are sets and repetitions? Are you totally lost? That's okay. I'm
going to give you a free pass; since you don't understand, you can
choose not to work out. Believe me? Of course not—you know I
don't let anyone off easy. After all, I want you to succeed!

Your lifting schedule will be the one given on page 127. All you
need is a little knowledge on how to do each lift and which lift
works what body part. Get ready to get smart. When I went
through this drill with my own family, I actually gave each person a
pen and when I asked, "Who knows where the biceps is?" one person would write "biceps" on someone else's arm. It was a great drill
that forced them to learn where their muscles were while getting a
good laugh at each other's expense.

Here are the body parts that you are going to work out:

Chest: The chest is the area between your neck and your
  stomach.
Biceps: Hold out your hand as if someone were going to give
  you something. The top of your arm in that position is your
  biceps.
Triceps: Hold out your hand as if someone were going to give
  you something. The back of your arm in that position is your
  triceps.
Shoulders: Lean your head all of the way to the right and the
  left until it touches something; that is your shoulder muscle.
Back: Your back muscles extend from your waist to your
  shoulders.
Quads: the top front part of your leg.
Hamstrings: the top back part of your leg.
Calves: the lower back part of your leg.
Abdominals: your stomach, from your chest to your waist.

Now, for sets and repetitions. You complete a set by repeating an exercise motion ten times. For example, if you are working out your shoulders on a shoulder-press machine, you do each movement ten times, rest for a minute, do ten again, rest again for a minute, and do a final ten repetitions. You have just done three sets of ten repetitions. Look, you're learning the lingo. Once you've completed your shoulder workout, move on to another body part and follow the same pattern.

You can do hundreds of exercises for each body part. The goal is to continue to learn new ones all the time. Experiment with your body to find exercises that you can do comfortably. If something feels good, then keep on doing it; if it doesn't feel good, then don't do it.

Let's say that today is your first weight workout and you decide to start with your triceps. Undoubtedly you are thinking, What in the world should I do? I have two suggestions to help you find your first triceps exercise. First, ask the gym staff. They will almost always agree to help you do it the right way. They may show you an exercise using free weights or how to use one of the resistance machines.

As you test resistance machines either by yourself or with a staff member, pay attention to the directions printed on the equipment: almost all feature a picture of a guy using the machine with a part of his body highlighted in red. Find a machine with the triceps highlighted and then do exactly what the picture on the machine shows you to do. It won't take long before you are very proficient and have compiled a list of three or four different exercises for each body part.

The second suggestion is to go to one of my favorite websites, http://www.bodybuilding.com/fun/exercises.htm. There you will see some enormous bodybuilders with arrows pointing to their body parts. Clicking on the links will take you to a website with pictures of lifting exercises and a video showing you how to do them properly. Although these are bodybuilders, they are doing the same exercises you are going to be doing. Use this valuable resource to add variety to your workout.

Don't expect to do resistance training right the first time. Just do a little better today than you did yesterday—and you will do fine.

WORKING OUT AT THE GYM AT HOME

Maybe going to the gym is not your thing and you have gym equipment and free weights at home. Great! It doesn't matter where you work out as long as you do something that you can track. The variety of machines the gym offers is a big plus, but working out at home is perfectly fine.

Not everyone can afford a gym membership or expensive gym equipment. In fact, for some it may have been a stretch to buy this book. I want to share my secret for buying or financing high-quality gym equipment at a superlow price. I recently bought a $2,500 Bowflex machine with all the attachments, in perfect shape, for $300. I know people who buy treadmills for $50 to $100, and there's a lot of affordable equipment if you know where to look. Here is the secret: everyone in the world (except you) has a treadmill, Bowflex, cross-trainer, or stationary bike in the basement gathering dust that they always think they are going to use but never touch. They bought it one day when they were motivated to get healthy and instead used it as a clothes hanger or storage space. Here's a funny e-mail I sent to our group of one hundred volunteers:

> As many of you know, my business requires me to spend a lot of
> time in other people's houses, and if I have noticed one thing
> about mankind it is this: almost everyone has a treadmill or a
> Soloflex in their basement that they have never touched. Usu-

ally, this item becomes a storage platform for boxes and old clothes.

This is why I wanted to announce this special congratulation to Colene M, who by the way has lost 12.4 lbs so far. This week she had a wonderful thing happen. This is the e-mail she sent me:

Tony,
Do you know anyone who services treadmills, or the best place to contact for repair? My treadmill quit working on the incline last night in the middle of my workout.

Colene M

Colene, your treadmill didn't break, YOU BROKE IT! And for that you should be proud. That's right, while the rest of the world is using their exercise equipment for storage, all of us are working our machines until they are pleading for us to stop and smoke is pouring out of the engine. Finally something has to give; the machine makes the decision that it will never beat YOU, and it gives up! Way to go, Colene!

If anyone wants to send condolences to Colene concerning her machine, send them to me and I will forward them. Also, if anyone knows a treadmill doctor who might be able to revive her machine, let me know.

Keep it up everyone!

TD

A lot of people really do have a machine sitting around gathering dust. So instead of wishing you had some good equipment, try to find some. Make a flyer: "Looking for cheap gym equipment that needs a good home. I am getting in shape, but I don't have money to spend at the gym. If you have anything you want to get rid of or sell cheap, please call me at 555-5555."

If you put flyers in thirty doors, you'll get so many calls that you won't know which piece of equipment to buy. Plus, this is the one day I will count walking as exercise! See how flexible I am?

If you are low on cash when somebody calls, that's okay. Look at the machines and make an offer: "I know you want $900, but would you take $300?" Remember, they are getting nothing now, and sometimes people just want to get rid of their old stuff, so they'll say yes to a lower price. If you are really short on cash, ask if they will accept $50 a month. After all, this is much better than what they were getting when the machine was gathering dust. In no time you'll be able to create your own little gym at home.

YOU CAN DO MORE THAN YOU THINK

Finally, there is just one more thing I want to say about exercise. The human body is much stronger than you realize. You can do much more than you think you can, and that is why you can accomplish so much more when you have a trainer or a workout partner pushing you. Once you start working out consistently and your muscles feel the strain of resistance, your mind is going to try to trick you into thinking that the training is just too hard for you. You will want to quit. But when you feel that way, consider it the signal that you are on the right track.

It really does take some time to get used to exercising and lifting weights consistently, but it doesn't take long. Within a couple of weeks, you will notice that those old, ragged muscles don't feel so stiff anymore, and you will enjoy the feeling that you get from doing regular cardio workouts and weight lifting. But to get there, you have to stop whining about it being hard and give it your all. Don't listen to that little voice that says, "It's too hard." You must overcome the human urge to quit and instead press forward.

Hire a trainer who will push you to the limit if you can afford it. If you can't, team up with someone and push each other. Do some research and learn the ropes together. Choose your resistance exercises together: you can pick a triceps workout and your teammate can pick one for the biceps. Teach each other how to do the exercise to the best of your ability. Neither of you will be perfect, but as you continue to try new lifts, you will improve. You will notice what other people at the gym are doing and say, "Hey, let's try that." It won't happen overnight. Concentrate on what you are doing today so that you can improve next time.

After just a few workouts, you will notice that your muscles feel stronger, lifting things will be easier, and many of your aches and pains will go away. The human body is a strong and powerful machine constructed for hard work, not for sitting in front of a computer all day. Work out vigorously–your body will love you for it!

Remember
- Exercise every day–no exceptions!
- Do two days of resistance training.
- Do five days of cardio for thirty to sixty minutes.
- Focus on improvement every time.

Chapter 8

WEEKLY WEIGH-INS, DAILY CHECK-INS, AND OTHER TOOLS OF ACCOUNTABILITY

People always ask me, "What is the secret to the F.A.S.T. diet?" This chapter is the secret. If you use the knowledge you have learned so far and then apply it using the principles of accountability this chapter offers, you will succeed.

Before I share how the accountability works, you need to understand why it is so critical to you and your success dieting. We all know that being overweight is bad and has life-threatening consequences. In fact, we know all kinds of things are bad for us, like smoking, drinking, doing drugs, stealing, and lying. Now for the kicker: not only do we know these behaviors are bad, but we know how to stop them. To quit smoking, all you have to do is stop putting those cancer sticks in your mouth. To stop drinking, you don't buy alcohol and don't consume it. The secret to losing weight is also well known: diet and exercise. Most of us can even act on these solutions and succeed for a couple of days. But how do you stretch those days into weeks and then years? The secret to the F.A.S.T. diet is to create an environment that turns a couple of days of success into a lifetime by relying on accountability to sustain constant motivation.

Creating and maintaining accountability around the team concept is the real magic behind the F.A.S.T. diet. It really is the reason we have had such huge success when everyone else is failing so badly. When people diet, they often feel that, no matter how hard they try, they can't win. It seems impossible. They fail every time they try.

Fortunately, accountability solves this problem. How? By creating another problem. Accountability makes most people feel uncomfortable. It is not fun to be held accountable when all you really want to do is eat a huge bag of M&M's at the movies. Accountability is definitely not fun when everyone is drinking on New Year's Eve and you're still sober. But let me ask you this: would you give up drinking on New Year's Eve or eating candy for the rest of your life if you could push a button and instantly have the perfect body, perfect health, and enough energy to do all the things you've been putting off for years? Most people would say yes. Fortunately, you don't have to give up those things forever—just for a year. Once you reach your weight-loss goal and are maintaining, making those exceptions a couple of times a month will not hurt you at all. In fact, when you realize that you can have fun and go overboard once in a while and still maintain your weight and be in control, you'll be more confident.

So, my point is this, you will only love the accountability once you have succeeded. While you are in the middle of it, it makes your life a little harder, but it is exactly what you need to succeed. The team is the most important tool of accountability. Here are a few others:

WEEKLY WEIGH-IN

The weekly weigh-in is a critical element to success on the F.A.S.T. diet. To make your weigh-in successful:

- Weigh in at the same day and time every week. My family chose Saturday at 8:15 a.m.
- Weigh in at the same location. Try to pick a central location that's convenient for everyone who will attend. The person hosting the weigh-in will need to be flexible. From time to time someone on your team will call and say something like "Hey, Julie. I need to miss this week's weigh-in because my kids have a basketball tournament." Missing weigh-ins is *never* acceptable: it is the team's responsibility to come up with a solution: "No problem. What time is the game? How about coming over to weigh in at six in the morning?" I have had people weigh in at my house at 4:30 a.m.–I'm not joking–not because I wanted to, but because as soon as you allow people to miss weigh-ins the accountability factor is completely shot. Your teammates will know that if they've had a bad week, all they have to do is make some excuse why they can't weigh in and they won't be held accountable. And, believe me, that is exactly what will happen.
- Use the same scale every week. From the first weigh-in on, no one ever gets to weigh in on any other scale except this one. *Never!* Also, no one can weigh in on any other days except the weigh-in day one time per week–no exceptions.

  When we started the F.A.S.T. program, my family weighed in one time a week just like I am telling you to do. However, I weighed in every day for nine months so that I could track how my body responded to the F.A.S.T. program. The results were unbelievable. I would start a week at 180 pounds and after a hard week of exercise and eating right, I would end at 178 pounds. This pattern was very consistent.

If you looked at my weight loss on a weekly basis, it seemed like success and it was. But if you looked at it on a daily basis, the numbers were all over the board. On day 1, I was 178 pounds; on day 2, I was 181, even though I was doing all the right things. On day 3, I was 177, 175 on day 4, and so on. The problem came when I weighed myself on that high day. Everyone's weight fluctuates from day to day. If you accidentally weigh in on a high day, suddenly you feel like a failure. If you weigh in on a day when your weight stays the same, you feel like a failure because you are not losing. If you weigh in on a very low day, you feel great, but then at the end of the week when your weight is a little higher but still 2 pounds lower than it was at the start of the week, you feel like a failure again, even though you have lost 2 pounds. Weighing in every day is diet suicide. Don't do it; fight the urge. Only do it if you want to fail—trust me.

■ Weigh in in front of as many people as possible. At first, your teammates will be very hesitant to do this because they don't want others to know how much they weigh. It is much easier if you all do it together—that way everyone is vulnerable together. The best part is that weigh-ins become fun after the first week. People get very excited when they lose weight, and when everyone is losing, things get downright chaotic— it's lots of fun. Our Omaha group weighs in on Saturday mornings and includes more than thirty people. As soon as the first person stands on the scale, the gathering starts to look like a wedding reception instead of a diet weigh-in. The person hosting the weigh-in must also wait to weigh in him- or herself until the group arrives. Everyone must be held accountable.

Include as many people as possible. Bring your family, kids, and friends if they want to come. Everyone gets to see how much you weigh that week. The purpose isn't to embarrass anyone but to help people realize and acknowledge that they have a problem. It's easy to lie to yourself in private, but in public there is simply no way you can lie anymore. When you stand on that scale and everyone hears that you are now 334 pounds, you will release a huge sigh of not only disgust and embarrassment but also relief. There's no more need to lie, fib, or hide. The only thing left to do is to prove next week that your days as a fatty are over.

When someone is about to step on the scale for the first time at our Omaha group weigh-in, I ask him or her, "How much do you think you weigh?" Every time the scale shows a number higher than the answer I'm told. Without exception, the person will say, "Wow, I can't believe I weigh that much." Later, sometimes even weeks later, he or she admits, "I actually knew I was that heavy. I was just afraid to admit it. In fact, I weighed myself a couple of hours before I came to your house." This is why a group weigh-in is so important. It forces you to acknowledge the truth and deal with it. Clarity in thought and purpose is power.

At my family's first weigh-in, my father and mother were both shocked by their actual weights. I asked my father how he would rank his health on a scale of 1 to 10. At five feet six inches tall, fifty-nine years of age, and 274 pounds, he answered, "About a seven." Today he is 170 pounds, and I recently asked him how healthy he thought he was back then. He said about a 3. I reminded him of his earlier answer, which I happened to have on videotape, and he was amazed. He had been lying to himself. This is a great lesson because we all do this. We have a tendency to make things seem better than they actually are, especially when it involves our own inadequacies.

A very intelligent mentor of mine who is a successful business-man once told me, "You can't change a lie." It is so true; you can't change who you are until you stop lying to yourself. If you quickly skimmed through that last sentence, *stop, pause,* and then reread it. Anytime you are trying to improve yourself in any way, the first thing you need to do is *start telling yourself the truth.*

For my family, our moment of truth came when we weighed in after having been on the F.A.S.T. diet for one week.

Everyone had been working hard, eating right, and holding each other accountable. I was sitting with my wife Friday evening talking about everything that had happened and then it hit me like a sledgehammer: what if no one lost any weight? After all, who was I? I was certainly no doctor. I wasn't a nutritionist nor a personal trainer. Was it really possible for an ordinary guy to create a simple system that would help a group of people, who probably had fifty failed diets in their past, lose weight? I had never felt this much stress and tension. We talked some more and then with much diffi-culty I finally got to sleep.

On Saturday morning I woke up about 7:00 to prepare for the weigh-in at 8:15. Everyone showed up on time and no one brought their kids. I gave everyone a quick pep talk and said, "There is no telling what will happen this first week. We could all have gained five pounds. Whatever happens, don't panic." We really had no clue.

My dad was the first one to step on the scale. The scale was in an upstairs bathroom so it was just him and me in the room. Every-one else was outside the door waiting to hear the results. As he stood on the scale, the numbers jumped around a bit, and I said, "Dad, quit moving and stand up straight." Finally the number stabi-lized; he had lost 12.5 pounds. I went crazy! "Dad lost 12.5 pounds!"

I screamed. Then everyone went insane: jumping up and down, crying, screaming, yelling. I was surprised that a neighbor didn't call the police. I'm not kidding. It sounded like a combination of Mardi Gras and Carnival. My dad had lost almost two times as much as an average newborn weighs at birth.

Mom was next. Could Dad's results have been a fluke? Dad stepped off the scale and walked out to high fives and hugs. Mom walked in. Looking at her face you would have thought we were just about to remove her appendix. She was extremely nervous when she stepped on the scale. She was trying to look down to see the numbers (skinny people don't understand that we fatties can't always see our feet without bending over), so I said, "Stand up straight." The numbers stabilized again . . . 252. I quickly did the math. "Mom lost thirteen pounds," I screamed.

Suddenly there was chaos again—we realized that the F.A.S.T. diet worked. The first week the eight of us lost a total of 67.5 pounds. Losing weight as part of a team is so much more rewarding than trying to be the Lone Ranger and go it alone. Tracy lost the least amount that day: 5 pounds. She was the lightest of the group, so that made sense. Because Tracy was part of the team, she was not too concerned about her last-place finish; instead, she was thrilled that she was part of the big number . . . 67.5 pounds. She was on the winning team now!

From that point on we were an unstoppable train, and our weekly weigh-ins became an opportunity to share our successes and celebrate.

By the third week, we had lost more than 100 pounds. As the changes took place, no one kept any of them secret. My dad started tying his shoes *on his own*. I know, this sounds easy, right? No! Not for a fatty. My mom would actually tie my dad's shoes because he could not bend over to do it. Now he could tie his own shoes and see his feet. I remember him saying, "Wow, this is new, I can see my

The Night Before: How to Prepare for a Weigh-in

- Consume all of your food and drink for the day before 8:00 p.m.
- Stay away from foods that are high in sodium and don't salt your food (the more salt you eat, the more water weight you will retain).
- Do not work out later than 10:00 p.m. and do not work out before the weigh-in tomorrow.

By the time you wake up, you will be thirsty and hungry and your stomach will be ready for the weigh-in. If you keep the routine the same each week, you will have a much more consistent weight loss, because your stomach will always be empty before the weigh-in. From week to week you really will be comparing apples to apples. Get ready for your weigh-in tomorrow. It's probably going to be a good one.

feet when I look down." He knew that as a team member he needed to share this story with everyone. Pretty soon, a teammate's success was a source of pride for everyone. When Tracy was on the treadmill at midnight, she didn't complain, because she was not going to be the one who let her dad down. His success was everyone's success.

At one weigh-in, each of my sisters pulled out her pair of "skinny jeans." I'm sure you know exactly what I'm talking about or you wouldn't be reading this book—that pair of jeans you used to wear in high school that you just can't get rid of because you hope to wear them again someday. My sisters were all wearing theirs and everyone knew it.

It was a very happy time. We were all on cloud nine. Then disaster struck. In the middle of all this wonderful weight-loss success, we lost Tracy. . . . Yes, I'm serious: it was week 7–the family had lost 137.3 pounds and Tracy only weighed 136.8 pounds. *We had lost Tracy!*

"Losing" a family member became a goal each week. Almost as much as we were paying attention to our own weight, we were looking to see who was next. In week 8, we lost Tina. Our total loss that week was 156.3 pounds and Tina now only weighed 146.2 pounds. Pretty soon we lost Jamie and Julie and my parents and then there was no one left to lose. When we got to 400 pounds, I think someone said that we lost a lion. It was a fun time that wouldn't have been possible without the team and the accountability of a weekly weigh-in.

DIET LOG

You must fill out your diet log every day right before or after you eat or drink. You can't fill it out at the end of the day and hope that you didn't eat more calories than you should have. Put it in your purse, your desk, or wherever you need to so that it is available whenever you eat. Once you are done eating or before you start, enter the numbers in your log and total up your daily calories so far. This will help you to know how many calories you have left to eat at any point during the day. At the end of the day, you must total up all your numbers and add any exercise you did or vitamins you took. You keep yourself accountable by tracking what you eat and drink all day long: your goal is always on your mind.

When you go to your weekly weigh-in, it is your responsibility to look through each day of your partner's log. If either of you forgot to bring your log, leave the weigh-in immediately to retrieve it. The only reason teammates forget their logs is because they haven't been accurately recording their eating; they don't want you to see and then critique them. When this happens, they will often gain weight because they are guessing on food and when you guess, you always guess too low. Trading diet logs at weigh-in and checking them over promote good tracking habits that will hold you accountable and at the same time teach you about food. People who write down what they eat succeed at a much higher rate than those who do not.

DAILY CHECK-INS

Daily check-ins are the key to keeping you focused all week long; they make it possible for everyone to know when someone is struggling. Each day you must call your partner and review your numbers. Here's a sample conversation:

"Hi, Bill. How did you do yesterday?"

"Not bad, Mary. I had eight glasses of water. I ate 1,355 out of 1,400 calories, 21 grams of fiber, 71 grams of protein, and I did thirty minutes of exercise for 297 calories on the treadmill."

"Great job! Make sure you watch your fiber. Are you looking for foods that will get you above the twenty-five minimum?"

"Actually, I don't know what to do. Can you suggest anything?"

"Sure. Yesterday I found this cereal called All-Bran, and the fiber is 13 grams for 50 calories. I eat it each morning, and it helps me reach my fiber goal every day."

"Great idea. Thanks, I'll go buy some. How were your numbers?"

"Not bad at all. I had six glasses of water. I ate 1,212 calories out of 1,300, 31 grams of fiber, 77 grams of protein, and I did sixty minutes of exercise for 761 calories on the stair-climber."

"Nice exercise—way to go. Please make sure to drink your eight full glasses of water. When you exercise all the time, your body needs all eight glasses every day to operate at its highest level. The next time you are short water, will you make sure to drink the last two glasses before you go to bed?"

"Yes, I will."

"Sounds good. Have a great day tomorrow, and remember we are only three days from weigh-in, so call me if you struggle and need any help."

"Sounds great. Let's have an awesome day. Our next weigh-in is going to be fantastic."

The whole conversation takes about three minutes. During that time, you reconnect and realize you are part of something, and that feeling carries you through the next tough moment. After all, do you really want to call your partner and tell him or her that you are the weakest link in the group? No way. We all have a little pride. This is also the time to share ideas about food and exercise. Accountability leads to education.

If someone does not call and check in, it is because he is not ready, did terribly, or hasn't added up his numbers. If that happens, you need to call your partner right away to help. This is not a time to be accepting or to help someone make excuses; instead, be strong and hold him to his commitments. Helping your teammate and being strong when he is weak is what will make both of you succeed.

SHARE YOUR SUCCESS

Send E-mail

E-mail is a great tool for creating accountability. My family e-mailed each other to provide updates on our exercise records or just to motivate each other to keep at it. Those e-mails were a constant reminder that each of us was a part of something that was very serious but also lots of fun.

My dad learned how to e-mail while he was on the F.A.S.T. diet, and his updates were hilarious and very motivating:

> Add a record—the sit up bike, upright bike, sore butt bike, or whatever you want to call it: 60 minutes 520 calories.
>
> By the way, when I left the gym the guy at the desk asked me if I fell in the pool.
>
> Congrats to all the record breakers and holders.
>
> > CYA

Here's another:

> Well here is one for the books. As I was leaving the gym last night after doing an hour of torture on the cross trainer for 879 calories, with my gym clothes dripping with sweat, I walked by the guy at the desk as I was leaving and I said, "You should go down by the cross trainers and stop that guy from throwing buckets of water on people."
>
> What is even funnier is the guy at the desk looked!
>
> > CYA

Take Pictures

Take pictures each week and create a folder on your computer where they are dated and/or numbered.

My family did this from day 1, and we found that it was not only fun but very motivational. I have fifty-two weeks of my family's pictures. When we put them in order, the result is a flip chart that literally shows how each person disappeared. It is so fun to watch. I recommend buying a cheap digital camera if you can afford one. Take a picture each week from the same spot and in roughly the same lighting. As people get several months into the program, they will have tough times. It takes only a minute to send them their before and current pictures. This will help your struggling teammates visualize how much success they have had so far. When you see what you have accomplished with your own eyes, the hard days don't seem nearly as grueling.

Create a Website

Our website, www.thefastdiet.net, is one of our most effective tools of accountability. Almost everyone knows someone with computer savvy nowadays, and creating a simple website is very easy and cheap. Each week, after taking pictures, I posted them next to the initial "before" pictures so that everyone in our family could see them. As the Web address circulated, everyone was looking at the pictures, even all the aunts and uncles. This may scare you to death, and that's why you won't cheat when you really want to. No one wants to be a failure, especially for all the world to see. So, if you feel uncomfortable, that means you are probably doing the accountability thing *right*!

We also created a record board on the website. We decided to post a first-, second-, and third-place record for every machine at the gym.

Lifecycle 9500 HR Upright Bike
1. Tony Dean 564 Calories (Men's Record 7-31-06)
  2. Mike Dean 520 Calories (7-25-06)
  3. Tony Dean 507 Calories (7-14-06)
1. Jamie Sacks 314 Calories (Women's Record 1-20-06)
  2. Tina Chereck 309 Calories (7-13-06)
  3. Sheila Dean 266 Calories (7-13-06)

Elliptical

1. Tony Dean 1,077 Calories (Men's Record 12-31-06)
   2. Jeremey Wright 1,047 Calories (1-11-06)
   3. Tony Dean 985 Calories (12-17-06)
1. Tina Chereck 757 Calories (Women's Record 1-13-06)
   2. Tina Chereck 722 Calories (3-7-06)
   3. Nikki Dean 716 Calories (2-13-06)

The record board created accountability to constantly improve our workouts. At one point my brother, Jeremy, sent an e-mail to the group; he had burned 1,000 calories in sixty minutes. Up to that point, I had never done this, and I was in much better shape than he was. Jeremy's record broke the glass ceiling, and soon I burned 1,000 calories for the first time. Then my dad did it, and pretty soon the women started breaking this plateau. I used to think that 800 calories burned was an amazing workout, and now it barely causes me to break a sweat. If we had never created the record board, there would have been no reason to exceed our past efforts.

Another benefit of the record board was changing the way we used machines. Teammates were always looking for ways to max out the machines' capabilities to beat both themselves and the record holders. One day my sister Julie told me that she had done the treadmill at a 15 incline for one hour. I was shocked how was that possible? The machine would be practically sticking straight up in the air. If my little sister could do it, I had to assume I could, too. Soon the sweat was pouring off my face. I never would have attempted this had Julie not been trying to break a record. Instead she ended up proving that this new level of exercise was possible. I think it is a great idea to post your records on the fridge or somewhere where you will see them each day. Soon you will have an all-consuming passion to beat your last record. I call my favorite workout days "gazelle days." I don't know what causes them, but they're great. Most of the time when you exercise, you feel like you are really struggling just to get to the end, but every once in a while your body turns into a supermachine, and you feel like you could exercise all night and never get tired. It's so much fun. Continuous improvement in your fitness creates this phenomenon.

Video

I videotaped my family members for about an hour on the day we started the F.A.S.T. diet. I asked all kinds of questions about how they felt and why they wanted to get healthy. Over the course of the year, I created little movies combining the old video with new footage. "I can't even believe that was me" was the most common observation. The camera is a powerful tool. We even have a video of us all superfat on day 1, saying, "We are going to be on *Good Morning America*"–and then it actually happened! You know what they say: be careful what you wish for.

Be creative! Anything you can think of that will bring attention to both the successes and the failures will be a winner. Your imagination is the only limit to the different ways you can hold each other accountable. You can never have too much accountability: more times than not, people have too little. With all the temptations the world has to offer us, more accountability is almost always better.

Chapter 9

WHY DIETING IS HARDER FOR WOMEN: STRATEGIES FOR SUCCESS

I know what the men are thinking right now: traitor. Men, I totally understand; I felt the same way when I started the F.A.S.T. program. The truth is, no matter what you guys are thinking, I figured writing this chapter would get me bonus points with my wife.

Like most men, I have no clue about women in general. However, dieting for an entire year with five very strong, outspoken women changed all that. Before we began the program, I could always walk away from my sisters and my mother if I started to think they were acting a little crazy or emotional. But once the diet started, that all changed. I soon realized that I was not as smart about women as I thought I was.

Fortunately, and probably for the first time in my life, I started to think that maybe I didn't know everything, so I decided to see if I could learn from this experience. After all, if I ever hoped to be a good team captain and help the women in my family succeed, I would have to understand why they were doing what they were doing. This actually was not as hard as I expected it to be, because it soon became apparent that women and men share many characteristics, with just a few exceptions; however, those few exceptions make weight loss harder for women. This chapter is not designed to give you women an excuse but to teach you why you are working harder than the men in your group and how they are losing more weight. For the men, you need to learn compassion, because the truth is, when it comes to weight loss, we drew the long straw and they drew the short one. By the way, please don't confuse compassion with accepting excuses. The two are very different.

WOMAN ISSUE 1: WOMEN BURN FEWER CALORIES THAN MEN

The average woman is smaller and has less muscle mass than the average man. It is a mathematical fact that a forty-five-year-old man who is five feet eight inches tall and weighs 300 pounds needs 2,527 calories per day to maintain his exact weight. If he eats 2,027 calories per day and never exercises, he will be operating at a 500-calorie deficit. A 500-calorie-a-day deficit times 7 days equals 3,500 calories a week. Remember, 3,500 calories equals a pound of weight loss. So if this man eats 500 fewer calories a day, he will lose 52 pounds in a year without exercising.

On the other hand, a forty-five-year-old woman who is also five feet eight inches tall and weighs 300 pounds needs only 2,053 calories per day to maintain her exact weight. If she was to lower her calories, just like the man did, to 2,027, it would be a deficit of only 26 calories per day and she would lose only 2.7 pounds each year. That's right—this is not a misprint—the man would lose 52 pounds and the woman would lose 2.7 pounds. For the woman to lose 52 pounds like the man did, she would have to cut her calories to

1,553. Women, are you feeling angry? Sorry, but don't shoot the messenger.

Women also require a minimum of 12 percent body fat for their reproductive organs to function properly. Men only need 4 percent. Since women are generally smaller than men, they burn fewer calories throughout the day through metabolism and normal activity. Men, who are naturally larger, burn more calories both at rest and in motion. Finally, women have hormonal changes and their menstrual cycle to deal with. However you slice it, women get the short end of the dieting stick.

So what do you do if you are a woman? Easy—you deal with it, because there is nothing you can do but take solace in the fact that you are the better-looking and smarter species, and overcome this particular obstacle. You compensate by reducing your calories more than your male teammates need to (but stay above the safe level of 1,000 calories per day) and exercising your heart out.

Use this knowledge for good not evil. Use it to motivate yourself. Are you really going to let the world dictate your weight to you? Are you going to accept that just because you have a slight disadvantage you cannot succeed? No way! Work out harder, exercise longer, eat better, and track your numbers to perfection. Accept that your weight loss could take a little longer—just do a better job. Remember, you women can deliver babies, but we men can't even deliver our dirty clothes to the laundry basket. *Women are the strong ones.*

WOMAN ISSUE 2: TOM

During TOM (that time of the month), a woman becomes a water-storage tank (and water has weight). My sisters would always warn me when you-know-who was in town: "Aunt Flo is here" or "It's time for The Visit." Finally they settled on "Tony, bad news: TOM came to visit." Like most men, I would shrug and mumble "Whatever," but once we organized our Omaha group, I quickly realized that TOM was no excuse; it came with real drawbacks. Each week a few women would stand on the scale and their weight would stay the same; some would even gain weight. Sorry it took so long, women, but remember, we men are simple creatures.

Not understanding how TOM affects a woman's body is diet suicide for most women. Here is why. Let's say you are a woman who is dieting and doing everything perfectly. You work out thirty minutes a day and stay within your calorie limits; for three weeks in a row you lose weight. In the fourth week, TOM comes to town: you stand on the scale and see you have gained 2 pounds. Not to mention, you're a little irritable because you hate TOM and now he is messing with your diet. Where is your next stop? That's right, the supermarket, to pick up a pint of Ben & Jerry's. Good-bye diet, hello ice cream.

The good news is that the water gain is not real weight, and without it you probably would have lost a pound or two. Just keep on doing exactly what you should be doing: the following week, you will lose another pound or two and catch up. The week after TOM leaves, women who remain committed to diet and exercise will lose 2 to 4 pounds, or even more.

Several women in our Omaha group refused to have that bad week, so when they knew TOM was going to be stopping by, besides carving "I hate TOM" on their kitchen counters with a carving knife, they would step up their exercise that week and work even harder than they had before. They would refuse to make the excuse and found a way to overcome! Bravo, ladies. The solution to all weight-loss issues is always the same . . . overcome, overcome, overcome!

Believe me, I am not trying to say I understand every woman's body or how it will react to every situation; but I can tell you that I do know what seventy random women will do, and for the most part it is the same as the men. Eat right, stay below your daily calorie goal, exercise hard, and the weight will come off. If you cheat, don't measure food, and skip your workouts, you will find it twice as hard to lose weight.

Believe in yourself, because you can do it!

Chapter 10

NO EXCUSES: DIETING ON VACATIONS, HOLIDAYS, AND BIRTHDAYS

Whenever people think about dieting, events like vacations, holidays, birthdays, or even must-see-TV nights are used as excuses to procrastinate or cheat. People tell me the same things over and over, almost as if they are reading from a script, just in case they stumble across the motivation to get healthy.

"Oh, yeah, this year I'm going to lose eighty pounds. I have already decided that once I get past the holidays, I'm going to really start exercising and eating right."

How about this one: "My husband and I are going to Mexico this weekend, and when we get back, we're going to start dieting. We are both going to get serious this time and lose the weight."

One year before we started the F.A.S.T. program, my mother said, "Tony, you know what, this year I'm going to lose some weight. I'm just waiting for these next couple of birthdays to pass and then I'm going to get started." My mom recently did the math and found out why she never started: there are about 110 members of my family in Omaha alone, which means we have a birthday every three days. See the holes in this plan?

Eating cake and ice cream or anything else you want at a birthday party or celebration is perfectly fine. I love cake and I love ice cream. I sent Ben and Jerry an invitation to my wedding seven years ago; unfortunately, only Ben made it! However, if you are going to follow the F.A.S.T. diet plan, you need to prepare for these events so that you don't cheat. Save enough calories so that you can eat the cake and/or ice cream without going over.

Is food bad? Of course not; we need food. But your life, your vacations, and your decisions should probably not be made around something that will be flushed down the toilet forty-five minutes from now.

"Well, Tony, that's all great, but no matter what you say, I like to eat some cake on my birthday, and I like to eat a piece of pie on Christmas, and I love downing a couple thousand calories of Reese's peanut butter cups when my kids come back from trick-or-treating. No matter what you say, I enjoy it."

I understand. I used to feel the same way; really I did. But do you know why you like to do those things? Do you have any idea? Because that's what your parents did, that's what your friends do, and that's what you've always done. In addition to that, the media tells you to eat and drink merrily, so like sheep, you do exactly that. Don't take my word for it—check it out yourself.

Let's visit an alternate universe for a minute. Imagine for a second that you have a body like Brad Pitt's (for men) or Eva Longoria's (for women). You work out every day and are extremely healthy. You run stairs, chase your kids, and do anything else you want without ever getting winded or tired. Because your body is so healthy, you sleep soundly through the night and wake up feeling full of energy and vibrant. You have more than enough energy to accomplish everything you hope to each day. Imagine if you could make exceptions for vacations and holidays without the consequences you live with now. Wouldn't that be great?

In the real world, none of us is going to look like Brad or Eva, but anything is possible. And that is the way it is supposed to be. Unlike athletes and TV stars, we never get to enjoy a healthy body and make exceptions without serious consequences. Why? Because we never pay the price to get healthy *first;* instead, we make food exceptions first and then expect to get healthy second. It never works that way!

That reminds me of one of my favorite sayings: "Success demands payment up front; there is no layaway plan." People want to eat whatever they desire without exercising and still have a great body in excellent health. But it just doesn't work that way. You can make exceptions and you can take days off, but only *after* you have reached your goal weight and the level of health you are striving to achieve. If you make exceptions while you are losing weight, all you do is undermine the success you are having and slow down or stop your current progress. On the other hand, if you have some cake or take a week off for vacation and eat like a starving person when you are already healthy, the consequences are minimal. The following week you work out hard and you are right back to where you were. No big deal.

So this year, instead of making an exception for every birthday, every holiday, and every reason you can think of to cheat, don't cheat at all. For one year, build the foundation that will make your body a skyscraper instead of the old broken-down shack it has been in the past. Finally stop making exceptions for everybody else and do something *big* for yourself. Who says you have to eat chocolates on Valentine's Day? Hershey's, that's who. Instead of taking thirty seconds to pick up some chocolate that you will be paying for all week, why not do something that actually says "I love you," not "Here, enjoy this junk food."

VACATIONS

What about vacations, though? Surely you deserve to binge on vacation; after all, your life is very stressful and you worked really hard to earn it. Ladies and gentlemen, we all have stressful lives and we all have to work hard. Some of us have tough jobs and some of us have other issues in our lives that make them even harder, and, yes, we all need a vacation. But what does a vacation have to do with food?

Is it because the place you travel to has delicious food? Maybe, but isn't there delicious food everywhere? I'll bet that there are fifty restaurants within sixty miles of your house that serve better food than you will get on vacation and probably for less money, too. If it's all about the food, then why not stay close to home? I'll tell you why—because it's not a food issue.

"But, Tony, I want to be free on vacation and not feel restricted."

Tell me, how does gorging yourself on food help you do that? When you overeat, don't you feel slow and lethargic? Yes, of course you do. And doesn't overeating on vacation make you look like a trained seal in your bathing suit? It sure does. So how does food give you freedom? It doesn't.

I remember one trip that my wife, Nikki, and I took to Spain. We ate a lot of delicious food. We also took a few day trips, and one of them was to the enchanting city of Ronda. It was divided into two sections that were united by a beautiful architectural wonder built in 1735—a huge bridge built into the mountain that stretched across a gorge. Here is a picture:

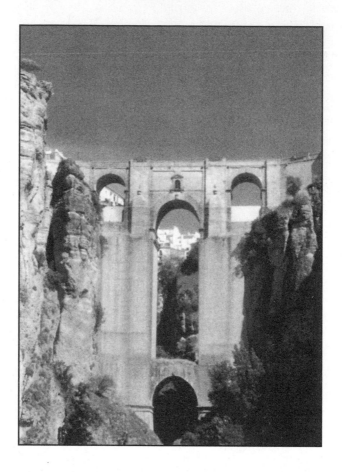

When we got home from that trip, what do you think we talked about first? "Mom and Dad, you have to hear about our trip to Spain. When we got there, we found this little restaurant where they served real Italian spaghetti that was delicious. Don't ask me why we ate Italian food in Spain, but it was amazing. We ate there three times, and each time, well, it tasted like...uh...spaghetti. And the Parmesan cheese, the flavor, it was amazing. It tasted like, well...Parmesan cheese. They also had this delicious bread, made of wheat and..." Actually, we didn't say a thing about the food. We pulled out pictures of that beautiful bridge and enchanting city, and we bragged for hours about how happy and lucky we were that we were able to see something like that.

All of us have been brainwashed by advertisers that food is fun and we need to spend lots of time and money to go to places and do things to get some special dish of food. To avoid this trap, you could purposely go on a vacation that is not centered around food. That would eliminate the temptation and make it much easier to stick to your diet on your trip. I don't think this is the answer, though, because the goal should be to make life changes for yourself, not to change the world to fit your lifestyle. Take advantage of what the world has to offer and enjoy it to its fullest, without being a slave to its vices.

How to Vacation on the F.A.S.T. Diet

First, don't change what you eat or the number of calories. There is no reason to eat more calories on vacation. Be active and do fun things; don't use food as a crutch. After all, you don't get to go on vacation every day, so live it up.

Write down everything you eat and drink in your diet log. Track everything, measure everything, and read labels. Remember, if you can't find the complete nutritional information for a food, *don't eat it*. This may seem strict, but strict is exactly what you need when you are losing weight. Remember, it won't be like this forever. Next year you will have a whole new body, and you'll have the choice to take a week off and recover the following week. But for this year, *no exceptions*. This is the year that you dictate your health, not Snickers or M&M's.

Your check-ins are also exactly the same. Before you go on vacation, set a time to check in with your partner or let him know when you will leave a message on his voice mail. Daily check-ins are a must: believe me, if you stop checking in, you will stop doing everything else as well. Remember, you won't have to do it on every vacation for the rest of your life—just this year. If you are traveling outside of the country, you should buy a phone card.

If you can be strong and fight off temptation while you are on vacation, that's great, but if you feel weak and are ready to do something you'll regret, call a team member and talk it out with him or her. Don't try to fight this battle alone—that's why you have been losing so far.

Exercise is the only thing that we do change. When you are on vacation, thirty to sixty minutes of uninterrupted activity counts as exercise. If your hotel has exercise equipment, then go ahead and use it. But you should also feel free to take advantage of your temporary environment. A long walk (or run) on the beach would be perfect. Take a paddle boat out for forty-five minutes and work your legs while you travel around the island and enjoy some remote spots that others might not get to see. Go scuba diving for an hour and swim and enjoy the underwater world. Volleyball, tennis, golf, and Jet Skiing are all fun, but do not count. Pick anything that will keep your heart rate elevated while you enjoy your vacation. For many people, their vacation workouts are some of the best and most enjoyable they will ever have. Try it. I guarantee that you will feel better and enjoy your vacation more. Most important, you will prove to yourself that this time nothing is going to stop you from losing weight successfully!

HOLIDAYS AND BIRTHDAYS

Many holidays seem to focus almost completely on food: Christmas, New Year's, Valentine's Day, Thanksgiving, even Easter and the

Fourth of July. On a holiday, feel free to eat anything you want, just not everything you want. Often it's easy for you because these meals offer healthy choices. For example, Thanksgiving turkey is great for you. But when you overeat, you turn a healthy meal into a diet bloodbath of rolls, gravy, and pie. Instead, plan for holiday meals, eat within your calorie limit, and then pat yourself on the back for keeping your success alive!

- Incorporate the F.A.S.T. diet into your celebration. We were all worried about how we were going to celebrate Christmas 2005 without breaking our diet. Our solution: each person was responsible for bringing a dish to the meal and a nutritional information card listing the calories, fat, carbs, fiber, and protein per serving size for everyone to take home and record in his or her diet log. We did the same thing for birthdays, Thanksgiving, and other holidays. We ate pie that year and all the foods we liked. Because we had all the numbers in front of us, we made sensible decisions instead of guessing.
- Plan ahead. If you plan to visit someone else's home for a holiday, explain the situation to your host and ask about the menu (as for restaurant dining, it helps to have the menu in advance). Or ask if you can help out and bring a dish or two to share. It's easy to overeat in a party atmosphere so don't arrive hungry. Have a light snack and drink plenty of water before the event so you'll be less likely to overindulge. Many times I will eat before I go and leave a little room for a small appetizer instead of a full meal.

Birthdays, vacations, and holidays are the hardest for most people. If you know that going in, then plan a little so you can have huge success and enjoy these occasions more than ever. If you are the partner of a person going on vacation, give him your all. Really push him because he needs you. Then when you go on vacation, he will be prepared to help you make it as well. This is no time for exception, this is the time for *excellence*.

Chapter 11

USING YOUR DOCTOR: BENEFITING FROM HIS OR HER EXPERIENCE AND KNOWLEDGE

Have you ever seen any book, advertisement, pamphlet, or anything else concerning exercise that did not finish with the phrase "Before starting any diet and exercise program be sure to consult your physician"? Me either. They all say it. In fact, I am certain that this book also has a disclaimer at the beginning, and in that sense it is much like other programs. But what is different this time is that I am going to teach you how to get your doctor on your team. I am going to teach you how to make his or her expertise work for you. Plus, I am going to show you how to use visits to your doctor as another level of accountability.

Is the last time you had a checkup too long ago to remember? Why? Because going to the doctor is no fun: he or she always wants to stick something in you, especially as you get older. "Hey, Doc, what's that little camera for?"—older men and women will know what I mean.

Despite all of this, your doctor needs to become your friend. It is time to recruit your doctor to join your team. I suggest that you get a checkup and ask your doctor for a copy of all your results. Learn the difference between good and bad cholesterol. Ask your doctor what you should do to get in shape and see if his or her recommendations coincide with what I am telling you to do. This will not only reinforce that you are getting good information but also give you some idea of your doctor's competency in these matters. Ask plenty of questions:

What is my ideal weight?

How many calories do I need to eat a day to maintain my weight?

How many calories should I eat to lose weight?

What exercises are best for someone my age to ensure long-term health?

Doctors are delighted when their patients decide to do something to improve their health. Many people think that doctors are pompous, rich jerks, but that hasn't been my experience. When you come in for your first examination after starting the F.A.S.T. program, your doctor will treat you like all her other patients. But three months later, when you return for your follow-up visit, she will ask you all kinds of questions: "John, this is great. Your resting heart rate is way down and you have lost thirty-five pounds. What are you doing?"

"Well, Doc, I started exercising every day with a group of friends, and we have lost 190 pounds together."

Suddenly your doctor will not be able to get enough of your success. Just recently, one of the new team members of our Omaha group lost 11 pounds in her first three weeks. Overweight since she graduated from high school, she was disabled and lived in Falls

City, Nebraska. It is one of those cities you can drive right by if you are not paying attention.

Lesle saw us on TV and sent me this e-mail:

> I am soooo interested in how this diet works. I have fought my weight all my life and I REALLY want to lose this time. I feel like I have a zipper at my throat and all I need to do is unzip and step out of this fat suit except the zipper is stuck.
>
>   I know you want people in Omaha, but I hope you will give me a chance. I need to lose at least 100 lbs. I am 5'3" and 250 lbs. 55 years old.
>
> Thank you,
Lesle
Falls City, NE

We laughed so hard while we were reading this e-mail, but we were inspired, and within three weeks Lesle was starting to get healthy. In addition to being disabled, she had type 2 diabetes. She had a close relationship with her doctor because she spent so much time in his office (for the most part because she was overweight). Three weeks after beginning the F.A.S.T. program, she went back to her doctor and he was stunned. He couldn't stop talking about how much better she looked; her entire attitude was better, and, best of all, her diabetes was gone. He wrote in big letters on her test results: DIABETES RESOLVED.

Before becoming involved in the F.A.S.T. program, I had no idea that diabetes had become a serious health crisis in our country. I simply did not pay attention. Then I noticed that many of the people in our Omaha group had it, especially type 2 diabetes, which is often controlled by diet and exercise. Time after time, people would start the program and before long their diabetes was gone. My father was one of them: he had type 2 diabetes; after he dieted and exercised consistently, it was gone.

As your health improves, you'll find that you can hardly wait for your next checkup. You jump on your doctor's scale, and he says, "Great job, Jim. You lost another seventeen pounds." Your response, of course, should be, "Doc, are you crazy? I think your scale is broken. I've lost 17.5 pounds. Here, let me take off my shoes."

There is another very important use for your doctor. He or she is the only person who can decide what you can and can't do when it comes to exercise. If you ever think that you can't exercise for a medical reason, call your doctor and ask him or her if that reason is valid. If your doctor says, "No, you can't exercise," then you are off the hook. But if he or she says it's okay to exercise, then you must do it. The decision-making process becomes very easy if you follow this rule. Almost always you will realize that you are making an excuse to get out of exercising and you will go to the gym.

Since you probably will be overweight and out of shape when you start the F.A.S.T. program, it's almost inevitable that you will injure yourself along the road to health. Your injury may be as simple as a pulled muscle or a bruise or as complex as a broken bone or a torn Achilles tendon like I had. Whatever it is, your doctor is the one who will decide if you can work out or not. If you are ever going to be a healthy person, you need to fight for your health.

Medical technology has advanced so much that doctors can pinpoint future problems long before they become serious; but the only way they can find them is if you stop by. Make it a goal to find ways to impress your doctor. Call your doctor every week if that is what you need to do. Physicians are in the "help people" business: they really do want to see you get healthy. All day long they deal with people who just want a pill to cover up their sickness but refuse to do anything to make a real change. You are like a breath of fresh air for your doctor.

Chapter 12

MAINTENANCE: ONCE YOU HAVE LOST IT . . . DON'T LOSE IT!

As you can imagine, we get a lot of questions about how to diet successfully:

"What do you eat?"

"Is it true that you don't eat any carbs?"

"I heard you never take a day off from exercising. Is that true?"

There is one question that I get asked often, and the bigger the person is, the more likely he or she is to ask it: "How exactly do you maintain the weight loss?" I have always thought that this was a ridiculous question for someone to ask at the beginning of the process because there is so much work to do and weight to lose before maintenance is even an issue. It is almost like doing financial planning before you have any money. Or going to court before anyone sues you. Or putting your leg in a cast before you have even broken a bone.

At the start of your diet, who cares how you are going to maintain the loss? At this point, all of your focus should be on getting to a point where you have something to maintain. Let's face it, most of us have never enjoyed the real pleasure of being healthy. Because of society's new MTV-video-game-never-leave-the-house-because-I-can-order-that-on-line lifestyle, many people have been fat all of their lives. Good health will be a cherished possession when you finally get it. When you are healthy, you realize very quickly that nothing is more important. Imagine that you had 1,000 pounds of gold bars. How would you protect them? What would you do to make sure someone didn't steal them from you? The answer is . . . *you would figure it out*. And when you finally get healthy using the F.A.S.T. program for losing weight, that is exactly what happens: *you really do figure it out*.

At this point, I am sure you are thinking, Tony, I have lost weight before and when I was done, I hadn't figured anything out. Instead, I almost immediately started gaining the weight back. Why is it different this time?

Because this time *everything* is different. When you get to the end of the F.A.S.T. process, when you need to start thinking about maintaining your loss, you will know so much more about food and exercise. You will be able to watch those late-night TV infomercials for the next fad diet and know exactly why it will or won't work. Your body won't feel the same way it did after your other diets; now it will actually feel *healthy*! Really healthy!

Remember, by this point you will have been exercising every day. Your heart will be a cardio machine. You will be able to sprint up a flight of stairs without breathing heavy, and maybe you'll try running in races, even marathons. Because you are working out so hard during the day, you will be tired at night (like you should be) and you'll sleep well and get the maximum benefits of sleep. You'll be eating much more fiber, and your body will have had plenty of time to flush out all the trash that was floating around in your system. Your body will have learned to live in a water-rich environment and will come to the conclusion that it will not have to starve or be deprived of what it needs to function at its highest levels. And don't forget, you will have been lifting weights. You won't look like Arnold Schwarzenegger, but your muscles will be much stronger.

The F.A.S.T. program is about much more than just losing weight. You will be healthy, and although I am about to give you instructions on how to maintain your weight loss, you will probably find out, like those who have succeeded before you, that the maintenance part will come very naturally. You will have attained a level of understanding about your body, exercise, and food that will not allow you to go back to your old habits.

Here's a maintenance-related pet peeve of mine. When I ask the question, "What would you like your goal weight to be?" people always answer it along the same lines: "I think I will shoot for 170 pounds, but I would like to be 150." I say, "What are you talking about? If you want to be 150 pounds, then let's get you to 150 pounds so you can enjoy your life the way that you have always wanted to; why even think about 170 at all?" Then we get to the root of the problem: "Well, Tony, I don't know if I can maintain 150 pounds."

Let me share a mathematical certainty with you: if you can maintain 170 pounds, you can maintain 150 pounds; most people need about the same amount of calories to maintain either weight. I can prove it. Remember the forty-five-year-old man and woman who each weighed 300 pounds? Sure you do. Let's say that the woman lost weight, and because she was scared that 150 pounds would be too hard to maintain, she stopped at 170 pounds.

At 170 pounds, she needs to eat 1,494 calories per day to maintain her weight. If she eats that much and does not exercise, she will never get fatter or thinner; she will maintain. On the other hand, if she drops to 150 pounds, her calories per day will change to 1,408, a difference of 86 measly calories: that means she has to give up three-quarters of a banana or one slice of bread each day. Big deal. But, hey, let's say that she wants to eat that slice of bread every day. When she finally reaches the maintenance phase, she will probably be able to burn those 86 calories in five minutes at the gym.

See what I mean when I say you should go for the weight you really want to be? I am telling you the truth. If you follow the F.A.S.T. program, you will be a changed person, with a new body and a huge repertoire of tools to help you stay fit.

Still don't believe me? That's okay; I wouldn't have believed it, either. When my family started reaching their goal weights, I created a weight-loss maintenance plan.

MAINTENANCE RULE 1:
MONITOR YOUR WEIGHT

Once you hit your goal weight, you still need to weigh in for the next three months with your group, but instead of going every week, you need to go only every other week. If you feel like you are regaining too much weight and are no longer comfortable, you must immediately reenter the program and check in with your teammate until you are back to your goal weight. You can choose to keep your diet log up to date: some people can't live without their diet logs and some people never touch theirs again. As long as you feel healthy and are satisfied with your current weight, do what feels best for you. My sister Tracy felt that she'd lost too much weight and decided to put a few pounds back on. If you find yourself above your goal and you aren't happy with your weight gain, you must start keeping track of everything again and reenter the F.A.S.T. program.

MAINTENANCE RULE 2:
CHOOSE A PERMANENT PARTNER

If you were rotating teammates during the weight-loss phase like my family did, you might have found someone you felt you could count on. That person should become your partner for life. That's right, I said for *life*. Once you are able to maintain your goal weight for three months, you must call your partner once a month and tell him or her how many pounds you weigh. Put a reminder on your calendar. If you are above your goal weight, you must reenter the F.A.S.T. program immediately to lose the unwanted pounds. What else makes sense? Did you begin this program so that you could be thin for a year or even a couple of weeks? No way—you were making this change for life. So, life it is.

MAINTENANCE RULE 3: INCREASE YOUR
CALORIES AND REDUCE YOUR EXERCISE

By now I am sure you understand how the mathematics of the F.A.S.T. diet work. It is really very simple. Remember when I told you to subtract 500 calories a day from your BMR number and those 500 calories a day would equal 1 pound lost per week? Here's the good news: you no longer have to do that. In fact, you now have to add calories or you will keep losing weight. Let's say your BMR number is 1,700 calories on the day you hit your goal weight, and you were eating 1,200 calories per day. Now that it is time to maintain, you need to move your calories back up to 1,700 per day (or whatever your BMR number is now that you are lighter and older). But surely you're not going to quit exercising, are you? You're not going to give up those wonderful feelings of being healthy, are you? No way.

Let's say that you have been burning 525 calories by exercising each day. I know that is hard to imagine now, but it won't be later. If you want to keep exercising that much, go ahead. Many people still exercise every day because they love the way it makes them feel, but a few people prefer to cut back to three or four times a week. Let's say you choose four days a week, which would equal 2,100 calories of exercise per week (525 × 4), which works out to 300 calories a day (2,100/7 = 300). That means you need to add 300 calories a day to your maintenance level of 1,700 calories per day, for a total of 2,000 calories to maintain your weight. If you eat less than that, you will lose weight. The whole process is wonderful: you get to exercise less and increase your calories to maintain.

The three rules discussed above are all you really need to know to keep your weight stable. Maintaining your weight will be much easier than you can imagine at the start of the F.A.S.T. program. You'll learn many things about diet and exercise to help you as you go along. It's true that we are all different, but despite our differences, we are still very much alike and share the same problems.

Writing this book is one of the most enjoyable things I have ever done. My eyes hurt from looking at the screen and my hands are sore from typing, but it doesn't matter, because I know that the F.A.S.T. program will benefit everyone who reads these words. It is a wonderful experience to have such a huge impact on so many people.

That being said, it is the individual successes that really make me feel like I am doing something big, and with your success, you will have the same opportunity. It won't be with your words but with your actions. Once you are up and running, I encourage you to say nothing to anyone other than your teammates during your weight loss, unless they ask. Instead, give everything to yourself and your teammates. When other people start asking you, "What have you been doing? Are you losing some weight?" go ahead and tell them everything; then offer to help them get involved. Become a mentor; captain their F.A.S.T. team.

Instead of just waking up and going to work each day and then coming home and watching reruns of *Seinfeld*, do something to make the world a better place. When you help just one person, that is exactly what you are doing. But you can't help anyone else until you help yourself, so get to work.

I recommend that you begin with the 10-Day Quick Start Program on page 175. I encourage you to enjoy the ride, be thankful for the advantages you have, and work hard. You were not meant to be overweight. Don't settle for being unhappy with your body. This time you actually are going to succeed!

Soon you will be healthier than you have ever been!

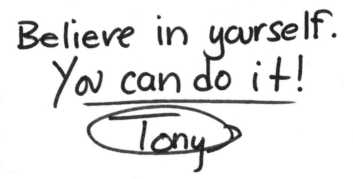

Be sure to send me an e-mail at tony@deanfast.com from time to time and tell me how you're doing.

10-Day Quick Start Program

It is time for the good news. You have read the entire book now and (I hope) had a few laughs. With any luck, you have learned a few things along the way, too. Anytime you take on a difficult project it is hard to figure out where you should start and then what you should do next. This day-by-day guide will help you get going.

DAY 1

- Weigh yourself.
- Finalize your team (see chapter 4). Choose your partner.
- Write in your diet log (see chapter 5 on tracking food and the diet logs starting on page 186) and have the totals finished by the end of the day. You can eat whatever you want, but make sure to write down everything you eat and drink and track the numbers exactly as you have been taught to do in chapter 5. The only food you cannot eat is anything for which you can't find the numbers of calories, carbohydrates, fats, protein, and fiber. If you can't find these numbers on the packaging, on the Web, or in a book or anywhere else, then you cannot eat that food.
- Don't forget to track any exercise you do. Fill in as much information on the diet log as possible.

■ Schedule a time to see your doctor. Make sure to discuss with him or her the changes you will be making in your diet and exercise routine.

DAY 2

■ Track everything you eat and drink in your diet log. Make sure you have everything totaled up before you go to bed that night. That's it. Easy.

DAY 3

■ As on days 1 and 2, track everything you eat and drink and add up the totals at the end of the day.
■ Prepare for your first official weigh-in tomorrow. Have you confirmed the place and time with your teammates?
■ Prepare for your first workout tomorrow (see chapter 7).
 • Have you secured a gym membership?
 • Or have you acquired gym equipment so you can work out at home?
 • If you have done neither, decide what exercises you will do.

DAY 4

■ Attend your first official weigh-in (see chapter 8).
 • Based on your current age, height, and weight, calculate your BMR using the formula on page 100 and determine how many calories you need to consume to lose weight. (Re-

member, never go below 1,000 calories for women and 1,200 calories for men.)

- Review the chart on page 102 and review how much fat, protein, and carbs you should consume daily.

■ Do your first workout. Exercise for at least thirty but no more than sixty minutes today and enter those numbers in your diet log (see chapter 7).

- Track everything you eat and drink in your diet log.
- Check in with your partner.
  - Did you stay within your calorie levels? Did your partner?
  - Did you eat at least 25 grams of fiber? Drink eight glasses of water?

DAYS 5–10

The following days will follow much the same pattern until you hit your goal weight:

■ Track everything you eat and drink in your diet log.

■ Work out. Try to beat yesterday's exercise numbers. Log your results.

■ Check in with your partner.

For a small percentage of people, day 5 is very hard because it is the second day your body has been eating at a calorie deficit. If you struggle, it is your job to call your teammate and ask for help: "Bill, I'm really hungry and I don't have any calories left; what should I do?" Let your teammate talk you through the problem. Utilizing your team is the secret to success, so make sure you use yours.

■ Resist the urge to weigh yourself before the weigh-in!

■ On day 10, prepare for the weigh-in the next day.

DAY 11

- Weigh in. Three things may happen during this weigh-in:
  - You will lose 1.5 to 5 pounds. This is the result most people will have, and if this is you, then congratulations. You obviously are doing great and are following the program like a champ. Keep improving each day and you will continue to see big results.
  - You will lose a huge number, from 5 to 15 pounds. My parents lost more than 12 pounds each their first week. Needless to say, they were a little surprised. If this is you, congratulations, but you need to mentally prepare for the fact that *this will not continue.* And you really don't want it to. In the following weeks, your goal should be to lose 1 to 2.5 pounds per week, and if you exercise and eat like you have been, you can almost expect it like clockwork.
  - You will gain weight or lose less than a pound. This result is extremely rare if you are following the program, but it does happen. You need to go through your diet log again and make sure you are not estimating numbers. Double-check how you are measuring quantities. If you are guessing and saying things like "a cheeseburger is about 500 calories," then you will fail. You *must* be exact. Also, if you are eating less than the minimum amount of calories per day, your body may go into starvation mode and drastically lower your metabolism; as a result, you won't lose weight. But if you have done everything right and you still didn't lose, then don't worry. Keep your focus and the following week you will see a great loss.

Finally, no matter what you do for the rest of the day, don't celebrate your weight loss with food. Keep your focus, stay below your calories, and work out harder today than you did yesterday.

Don't forget, today you still need to:

- Track everything you eat and drink in your diet log.
- Work out. Try to beat yesterday's exercise numbers. Log your results.
- Check in with your partner.

Now you know everything you have to do to lose weight. Follow this routine and prepare for a wild ride to health. You are going to be amazed at what happens over the next several months or several years, depending on how much you have to lose.

When people ask you why you seem more energized, tell them our story and give them a copy of the book. When my family started this, we thought we might lose a few pounds and that would be the end of it; instead, every time we share our story, it seems that someone new is getting healthy. Now you can do the same thing. Your success will encourage and breed success in others. Instead of being part of the obesity epidemic, you become part of the solution.

You can do it!

Nutritional Values for Common Foods

Food or Beverage	Serving Size	Calories	Fat (grams)	Carbs (grams)	Fiber (grams)	Protein (grams)
Anchovies	3 oz	111	4.1	0	0	17.3
Apple (medium)	1	81	0.5	21.1	3.3	0.3
Applesauce (sweetened)	½ cup	97	0.2	25.5	1.5	0.2
Applesauce (unsweetened)	½ cup	53	0.1	13.8	1.5	0.2
Asparagus	1 spear	2	0	0.5	0.3	0.3
Avocado (medium)	1	306	30	12	4.7	3.6
Bacon (panfried)	2 slices	70	6	0	0	5
Bagel (plain)	1	150	1	34	1	9
Baked beans	½ cup	170	1	21	10.4	6
Banana (medium)	1	105	0.6	26.7	2.7	1.2
Beef (80% ground lean)	4 oz	308	20.9	0	0	28
Beef bologna	1 slice	88	8	0.6	0	3.3
Beef jerky	1	81	5.1	2.2	0.4	6.6
Blueberries	½ cup	41	0.3	10.2	3.5	0.5
Bratwurst	1	281	24.8	2.1	0	11.7
Broccoli	½ cup	12	0.2	2.3	1.3	1.3
Brownie	1	220	13	27	1	1
Butter	1 tbsp	100	11.4	0	0	0.1
Cake (yellow)	1 slice	260	11	36	1	2
Cantaloupe	½ cup	29	0.2	6.7	0.6	0.7

Food or Beverage	Serving Size	Calories	Fat (grams)	Carbs (grams)	Fiber (grams)	Protein (grams)
Carrot	1	31	0.1	7.3	2.0	0.7
Cashews (roasted)	18	163	8.1	13.7	1.1	4.6
Celery	1 stalk	6	0.1	1.5	0.7	0.3
Cheese (cheddar)	1 oz	110	9	1	0	7
Cheese (mozzarella)	1 oz	90	7	0.5	0	25
Chicken (dark meat)	4 oz	287	14	0	0	38
Chicken (light meat)	4 oz	196	5.1	0	0	35.1
Chili (with beans, canned)	1 cup	287	14	30.5	11	14.5
Chips (potato)	15	160	10	14	1	2
Coffee (brewed)	6 oz	4	0	0.8	0	0.1
Cookies (chocolate chip)	1	130	6.9	16.7	0.9	0.9
Corn (canned)	½ cup	80	1	17	2.1	2
Corn flakes	1 oz	100	0	24	1	2
Cottage cheese	½ cup	100	2	4	0	14
Crackers (Ritz)	5	80	4	10	0	1
Crackers (saltines)	1	20	1	4.1	0.1	0.5
Cucumber	1	45	0.3	10.9	1.5	2
Dill pickle	1	13	0	2.7	0	0.4
Doughnut (glazed)	1	250	12	33	1.4	3
Egg (raw)	1	75	5	0.6	0	6.3
Fish (cod)	3 oz	70	6	0	0	15.1
Fish (salmon)	3 oz	99	2.9	0	0	16.9
Frankfurter	1	174	15.8	1	1.4	6.6
French fries (frozen)	18	170	6.7	27.7	3.4	2.8
Grapefruit (medium)	½	46	0.1	11.9	1.4	0.6
Grapes (seedless)	10	36	0.3	8.9	0.3	0.3
Green beans (canned)	½ cup	22	0.2	4.9	2	1.2
Ham (lean, diced)	4 oz	249	12.5	0	0	32.1

Food or Beverage	Serving Size	Calories	Fat (grams)	Carbs (grams)	Fiber (grams)	Protein (grams)
Ice cream (vanilla)	½ cup	144	7.9	16.9	0.5	2.5
Jelly	1 tbsp	56	0	13.8	0.2	0.1
Lettuce (shredded)	½ cup	5	0.1	1	0.5	0.4
Mac & cheese	1 cup	410	18.5	48	1	11
Maple syrup	1 tsp	50	0	13	0	0
Mayonnaise	1 tsp	100	11	0	0	0
Milk (2%)	1 cup	138	4.9	13.5	0	9.7
Noodles (egg, cooked)	1 cup	212	2.4	39.7	1.8	7.6
Oatmeal (uncooked)	½ cup	150	3	27	4	5
Orange (navel)	1	65	0.1	16.3	3.1	1.4
Orange juice	6 oz	80	0	20	0.1	0
Pancake (buttermilk)	1	86	3.5	10.9	0	2.6
Pasta (cooked)	1 cup	197	0.9	39.7	2.4	6.7
Peach	1	37	0.1	9.7	1.7	0.6
Peanut butter	2 tbsp	188	16	6.6	1.9	7.9
Peanuts (roasted)	1 oz	163	13.8	5.3	2.6	7.4
Peas (fresh)	1 cup	134	0.3	25	8.8	8.5
Popcorn (air popped)	1 cup	31	0.3	6.2	1.2	1
Pork loin	3 oz	199	11.4	0	0	22.3
Potato (baked)	1	220	0.2	51	4.4	4.7
Pretzels	1 oz	108	0.9	22.4	0.9	2.6
Rice (white, cooked)	1 cup	160	0.5	38	0	3
Roll (dinner)	1	136	3.1	22.9	0.8	3.6
Salad dressing (Italian)	1 tbsp	43	4.2	1.5	0	0.1
Salad dressing (Ranch)	1 tbsp	25	0	0	0	0
Salsa	1 cup	70	0.4	16.2	4.1	4
Shrimp (large, raw)	4	30	0.5	0.3	0	5.7
Soup (chicken noodle)	1 cup	75	2.4	9.3	0.7	4
Soup (vegetable)	1 cup	72	1.9	11.9	0.5	2.1
Strawberries	½ cup	23	0.3	5.2	3.3	0.5

Food or Beverage	Serving Size	Calories	Fat (grams)	Carbs (grams)	Fiber (grams)	Protein (grams)
Sugar (granulated, white)	1 tsp	15	0	4	0	0
Tomato	1	26	0.4	5.7	1.4	1
Tuna (canned in water)	2 oz	60	0.5	0	0	12
Turkey (light meat)	4 oz	178	3.7	0	0	33.9
Waffle (Eggo)	1	120	5	16	0	3
Watermelon (diced)	½ cup	25	0.3	5.7	0.4	0.5
Wheat bread	1 slice	70	1	12	1.4	3
Yogurt (plain, low fat)	1 cup	150	4	17	0	12

30-Day Diet Log

DAY 1

DATE: DAY OF WEEK:

WATER INTAKE: ○   ○   ○   ○   ○   ○   ○   ○

BREAKFAST	SERV	CAL	FAT	CARB	FIB	PRO	OTHER

LUNCH	SERV	CAL	FAT	CARB	FIB	PRO	

DINNER	SERV	CAL	FAT	CARB	FIB	PRO	

SNACK	SERV	CAL	FAT	CARB	FIB	PRO	

DAILY TOTALS		CAL	FAT	CARB	FIB	PRO	OTHER

EXERCISE	DURATION	INTENSITY	CALORIES BURNED

VITAMINS / QTY	SUPPLEMENTS / QTY	MEDICATIONS / QTY

DAILY JOURNAL

TODAY I FEEL:

DAY 2

DATE: DAY OF WEEK:

WATER INTAKE: ○   ○   ○   ○   ○   ○   ○   ○

BREAKFAST	SERV	CAL	FAT	CARB	FIB	PRO	OTHER

LUNCH	SERV	CAL	FAT	CARB	FIB	PRO	

DINNER	SERV	CAL	FAT	CARB	FIB	PRO	

SNACK	SERV	CAL	FAT	CARB	FIB	PRO	

DAILY TOTALS		CAL	FAT	CARB	FIB	PRO	OTHER

EXERCISE	DURATION	INTENSITY	CALORIES BURNED

VITAMINS / QTY	SUPPLEMENTS / QTY	MEDICATIONS / QTY

DAILY JOURNAL

TODAY I FEEL:

DAY 3

DATE: DAY OF WEEK:

WATER INTAKE: ○   ○   ○   ○   ○   ○   ○   ○

BREAKFAST	SERV	CAL	FAT	CARB	FIB	PRO	OTHER

LUNCH	SERV	CAL	FAT	CARB	FIB	PRO	

DINNER	SERV	CAL	FAT	CARB	FIB	PRO	

SNACK	SERV	CAL	FAT	CARB	FIB	PRO	

DAILY TOTALS		CAL	FAT	CARB	FIB	PRO	OTHER

EXERCISE	DURATION	INTENSITY	CALORIES BURNED

VITAMINS / QTY	SUPPLEMENTS / QTY	MEDICATIONS / QTY

DAILY JOURNAL

TODAY I FEEL:

DAY 4

DATE: DAY OF WEEK:

WATER INTAKE: ○ ○ ○ ○ ○ ○ ○ ○

BREAKFAST	SERV	CAL	FAT	CARB	FIB	PRO	OTHER

LUNCH	SERV	CAL	FAT	CARB	FIB	PRO	

DINNER	SERV	CAL	FAT	CARB	FIB	PRO	

SNACK	SERV	CAL	FAT	CARB	FIB	PRO	

DAILY TOTALS		CAL	FAT	CARB	FIB	PRO	OTHER

EXERCISE	DURATION	INTENSITY	CALORIES BURNED

VITAMINS / QTY	SUPPLEMENTS / QTY	MEDICATIONS / QTY

DAILY JOURNAL

TODAY I FEEL:

DAY 5

DATE:				DAY OF WEEK:			

WATER INTAKE: ○ ○ ○ ○ ○ ○ ○ ○

BREAKFAST	SERV	CAL	FAT	CARB	FIB	PRO	OTHER

LUNCH	SERV	CAL	FAT	CARB	FIB	PRO	

DINNER	SERV	CAL	FAT	CARB	FIB	PRO	

SNACK	SERV	CAL	FAT	CARB	FIB	PRO	

DAILY TOTALS		CAL	FAT	CARB	FIB	PRO	OTHER

EXERCISE	DURATION	INTENSITY	CALORIES BURNED

VITAMINS / QTY	SUPPLEMENTS / QTY	MEDICATIONS / QTY

DAILY JOURNAL

TODAY I FEEL:

DAY 6

DATE: DAY OF WEEK:

WATER INTAKE: ○   ○   ○   ○   ○   ○   ○   ○

BREAKFAST	SERV	CAL	FAT	CARB	FIB	PRO	OTHER

LUNCH	SERV	CAL	FAT	CARB	FIB	PRO	

DINNER	SERV	CAL	FAT	CARB	FIB	PRO	

SNACK	SERV	CAL	FAT	CARB	FIB	PRO	

DAILY TOTALS		CAL	FAT	CARB	FIB	PRO	OTHER

EXERCISE	DURATION	INTENSITY	CALORIES BURNED

VITAMINS / QTY	SUPPLEMENTS / QTY	MEDICATIONS / QTY

DAILY JOURNAL

TODAY I FEEL:

DAY 7

DATE:				DAY OF WEEK:			

WATER INTAKE: ○   ○   ○   ○   ○   ○   ○   ○

BREAKFAST	SERV	CAL	FAT	CARB	FIB	PRO	OTHER

LUNCH	SERV	CAL	FAT	CARB	FIB	PRO	

DINNER	SERV	CAL	FAT	CARB	FIB	PRO	

SNACK	SERV	CAL	FAT	CARB	FIB	PRO	

DAILY TOTALS		CAL	FAT	CARB	FIB	PRO	OTHER

EXERCISE	DURATION	INTENSITY	CALORIES BURNED

VITAMINS / QTY	SUPPLEMENTS / QTY	MEDICATIONS / QTY

DAILY JOURNAL

TODAY I FEEL:

DAY 8

DATE:				DAY OF WEEK:			

WATER INTAKE: ○　○　○　○　○　○　○　○

BREAKFAST	SERV	CAL	FAT	CARB	FIB	PRO	OTHER

LUNCH	SERV	CAL	FAT	CARB	FIB	PRO	

DINNER	SERV	CAL	FAT	CARB	FIB	PRO	

SNACK	SERV	CAL	FAT	CARB	FIB	PRO	

DAILY TOTALS		CAL	FAT	CARB	FIB	PRO	OTHER

EXERCISE	DURATION	INTENSITY	CALORIES BURNED

VITAMINS / QTY	SUPPLEMENTS / QTY	MEDICATIONS / QTY

DAILY JOURNAL

TODAY I FEEL:

DAY 9

DATE:				DAY OF WEEK:			

WATER INTAKE: ○ ○ ○ ○ ○ ○ ○ ○

BREAKFAST	SERV	CAL	FAT	CARB	FIB	PRO	OTHER

LUNCH	SERV	CAL	FAT	CARB	FIB	PRO	

DINNER	SERV	CAL	FAT	CARB	FIB	PRO	

SNACK	SERV	CAL	FAT	CARB	FIB	PRO	

DAILY TOTALS		CAL	FAT	CARB	FIB	PRO	OTHER

EXERCISE	DURATION	INTENSITY	CALORIES BURNED

VITAMINS / QTY	SUPPLEMENTS / QTY	MEDICATIONS / QTY

DAILY JOURNAL

TODAY I FEEL:

DAY 10

DATE: DAY OF WEEK:

WATER INTAKE: ○ ○ ○ ○ ○ ○ ○ ○

BREAKFAST	SERV	CAL	FAT	CARB	FIB	PRO	OTHER

LUNCH	SERV	CAL	FAT	CARB	FIB	PRO	

DINNER	SERV	CAL	FAT	CARB	FIB	PRO	

SNACK	SERV	CAL	FAT	CARB	FIB	PRO	

DAILY TOTALS		CAL	FAT	CARB	FIB	PRO	OTHER

EXERCISE	DURATION	INTENSITY	CALORIES BURNED

VITAMINS / QTY	SUPPLEMENTS / QTY	MEDICATIONS / QTY

DAILY JOURNAL

TODAY I FEEL:

DAY 11

DATE: DAY OF WEEK:

WATER INTAKE: ○　○　○　○　○　○　○　○

BREAKFAST	SERV	CAL	FAT	CARB	FIB	PRO	OTHER

LUNCH	SERV	CAL	FAT	CARB	FIB	PRO	

DINNER	SERV	CAL	FAT	CARB	FIB	PRO	

SNACK	SERV	CAL	FAT	CARB	FIB	PRO	

DAILY TOTALS		CAL	FAT	CARB	FIB	PRO	OTHER

EXERCISE	DURATION	INTENSITY	CALORIES BURNED

VITAMINS / QTY	SUPPLEMENTS / QTY	MEDICATIONS / QTY

DAILY JOURNAL

TODAY I FEEL:

DAY 12

DATE: DAY OF WEEK:

WATER INTAKE: ○   ○   ○   ○   ○   ○   ○   ○

BREAKFAST	SERV	CAL	FAT	CARB	FIB	PRO	OTHER

LUNCH	SERV	CAL	FAT	CARB	FIB	PRO	

DINNER	SERV	CAL	FAT	CARB	FIB	PRO	

SNACK	SERV	CAL	FAT	CARB	FIB	PRO	

DAILY TOTALS		CAL	FAT	CARB	FIB	PRO	OTHER

EXERCISE	DURATION	INTENSITY	CALORIES BURNED

VITAMINS / QTY	SUPPLEMENTS / QTY	MEDICATIONS / QTY

DAILY JOURNAL

TODAY I FEEL:

DAY 13

DATE: DAY OF WEEK:

WATER INTAKE: ○   ○   ○   ○   ○   ○   ○   ○

BREAKFAST	SERV	CAL	FAT	CARB	FIB	PRO	OTHER

LUNCH	SERV	CAL	FAT	CARB	FIB	PRO	

DINNER	SERV	CAL	FAT	CARB	FIB	PRO	

SNACK	SERV	CAL	FAT	CARB	FIB	PRO	

DAILY TOTALS		CAL	FAT	CARB	FIB	PRO	OTHER

EXERCISE	DURATION	INTENSITY	CALORIES BURNED

VITAMINS / QTY	SUPPLEMENTS / QTY	MEDICATIONS / QTY

DAILY JOURNAL

TODAY I FEEL:

DAY 14

DATE:			DAY OF WEEK:				
WATER INTAKE: ○ ○ ○ ○ ○ ○ ○ ○							
BREAKFAST	SERV	CAL	FAT	CARB	FIB	PRO	OTHER
LUNCH	SERV	CAL	FAT	CARB	FIB	PRO	
DINNER	SERV	CAL	FAT	CARB	FIB	PRO	
SNACK	SERV	CAL	FAT	CARB	FIB	PRO	
DAILY TOTALS		CAL	FAT	CARB	FIB	PRO	OTHER

EXERCISE	DURATION	INTENSITY	CALORIES BURNED

VITAMINS / QTY	SUPPLEMENTS / QTY	MEDICATIONS / QTY

DAILY JOURNAL

TODAY I FEEL:

DAY 15

DATE:			DAY OF WEEK:				

WATER INTAKE: ○ ○ ○ ○ ○ ○ ○ ○

BREAKFAST	SERV	CAL	FAT	CARB	FIB	PRO	OTHER

LUNCH	SERV	CAL	FAT	CARB	FIB	PRO	

DINNER	SERV	CAL	FAT	CARB	FIB	PRO	

SNACK	SERV	CAL	FAT	CARB	FIB	PRO	

DAILY TOTALS		CAL	FAT	CARB	FIB	PRO	OTHER

EXERCISE	DURATION	INTENSITY	CALORIES BURNED

VITAMINS / QTY	SUPPLEMENTS / QTY	MEDICATIONS / QTY

DAILY JOURNAL

TODAY I FEEL:

DAY 16

DATE: DAY OF WEEK:

WATER INTAKE: ○ ○ ○ ○ ○ ○ ○ ○

BREAKFAST	SERV	CAL	FAT	CARB	FIB	PRO	OTHER

LUNCH	SERV	CAL	FAT	CARB	FIB	PRO	

DINNER	SERV	CAL	FAT	CARB	FIB	PRO	

SNACK	SERV	CAL	FAT	CARB	FIB	PRO	

DAILY TOTALS		CAL	FAT	CARB	FIB	PRO	OTHER

EXERCISE	DURATION	INTENSITY	CALORIES BURNED

VITAMINS / QTY	SUPPLEMENTS / QTY	MEDICATIONS / QTY

DAILY JOURNAL

TODAY I FEEL:

DAY 17

DATE:				DAY OF WEEK:			
WATER INTAKE: ○ ○ ○ ○ ○ ○ ○ ○							
BREAKFAST	SERV	CAL	FAT	CARB	FIB	PRO	OTHER
LUNCH	SERV	CAL	FAT	CARB	FIB	PRO	
DINNER	SERV	CAL	FAT	CARB	FIB	PRO	
SNACK	SERV	CAL	FAT	CARB	FIB	PRO	
DAILY TOTALS		CAL	FAT	CARB	FIB	PRO	OTHER

EXERCISE	DURATION	INTENSITY	CALORIES BURNED

VITAMINS / QTY	SUPPLEMENTS / QTY	MEDICATIONS / QTY

DAILY JOURNAL

TODAY I FEEL:

DAY 18

DATE:				DAY OF WEEK:			

WATER INTAKE: ○   ○   ○   ○   ○   ○   ○   ○

BREAKFAST	SERV	CAL	FAT	CARB	FIB	PRO	OTHER

LUNCH	SERV	CAL	FAT	CARB	FIB	PRO	

DINNER	SERV	CAL	FAT	CARB	FIB	PRO	

SNACK	SERV	CAL	FAT	CARB	FIB	PRO	

DAILY TOTALS		CAL	FAT	CARB	FIB	PRO	OTHER

EXERCISE	DURATION	INTENSITY	CALORIES BURNED

VITAMINS / QTY	SUPPLEMENTS / QTY	MEDICATIONS / QTY

DAILY JOURNAL

TODAY I FEEL:

DAY 19

DATE: DAY OF WEEK:

WATER INTAKE: ○ ○ ○ ○ ○ ○ ○ ○

BREAKFAST	SERV	CAL	FAT	CARB	FIB	PRO	OTHER

LUNCH	SERV	CAL	FAT	CARB	FIB	PRO	

DINNER	SERV	CAL	FAT	CARB	FIB	PRO	

SNACK	SERV	CAL	FAT	CARB	FIB	PRO	

DAILY TOTALS		CAL	FAT	CARB	FIB	PRO	OTHER

EXERCISE	DURATION	INTENSITY	CALORIES BURNED

VITAMINS / QTY	SUPPLEMENTS / QTY	MEDICATIONS / QTY

DAILY JOURNAL

TODAY I FEEL:

DAY 20

DATE:			DAY OF WEEK:				
WATER INTAKE: ○ ○ ○ ○ ○ ○ ○ ○							
BREAKFAST	SERV	CAL	FAT	CARB	FIB	PRO	OTHER
LUNCH	SERV	CAL	FAT	CARB	FIB	PRO	
DINNER	SERV	CAL	FAT	CARB	FIB	PRO	
SNACK	SERV	CAL	FAT	CARB	FIB	PRO	
DAILY TOTALS		CAL	FAT	CARB	FIB	PRO	OTHER

EXERCISE	DURATION	INTENSITY	CALORIES BURNED

VITAMINS / QTY	SUPPLEMENTS / QTY	MEDICATIONS / QTY

DAILY JOURNAL

TODAY I FEEL:

DAY 21

DATE: DAY OF WEEK:

WATER INTAKE: ○   ○   ○   ○   ○   ○   ○   ○

BREAKFAST	SERV	CAL	FAT	CARB	FIB	PRO	OTHER

LUNCH	SERV	CAL	FAT	CARB	FIB	PRO	

DINNER	SERV	CAL	FAT	CARB	FIB	PRO	

SNACK	SERV	CAL	FAT	CARB	FIB	PRO	

DAILY TOTALS		CAL	FAT	CARB	FIB	PRO	OTHER

EXERCISE	DURATION	INTENSITY	CALORIES BURNED

VITAMINS / QTY	SUPPLEMENTS / QTY	MEDICATIONS / QTY

DAILY JOURNAL

TODAY I FEEL:

DAY 22

DATE: DAY OF WEEK:

WATER INTAKE: ○   ○   ○   ○   ○   ○   ○   ○

BREAKFAST	SERV	CAL	FAT	CARB	FIB	PRO	OTHER

LUNCH	SERV	CAL	FAT	CARB	FIB	PRO	

DINNER	SERV	CAL	FAT	CARB	FIB	PRO	

SNACK	SERV	CAL	FAT	CARB	FIB	PRO	

DAILY TOTALS		CAL	FAT	CARB	FIB	PRO	OTHER

EXERCISE	DURATION	INTENSITY	CALORIES BURNED

VITAMINS / QTY	SUPPLEMENTS / QTY	MEDICATIONS / QTY

DAILY JOURNAL

TODAY I FEEL:

DAY 23

DATE: DAY OF WEEK:

WATER INTAKE: ○   ○   ○   ○   ○   ○   ○   ○

BREAKFAST	SERV	CAL	FAT	CARB	FIB	PRO	OTHER

LUNCH	SERV	CAL	FAT	CARB	FIB	PRO	

DINNER	SERV	CAL	FAT	CARB	FIB	PRO	

SNACK	SERV	CAL	FAT	CARB	FIB	PRO	

DAILY TOTALS		CAL	FAT	CARB	FIB	PRO	OTHER

EXERCISE	DURATION	INTENSITY	CALORIES BURNED

VITAMINS / QTY	SUPPLEMENTS / QTY	MEDICATIONS / QTY

DAILY JOURNAL

TODAY I FEEL:

DAY 24

DATE: DAY OF WEEK:

WATER INTAKE: ○   ○   ○   ○   ○   ○   ○   ○

BREAKFAST	SERV	CAL	FAT	CARB	FIB	PRO	OTHER

LUNCH	SERV	CAL	FAT	CARB	FIB	PRO	

DINNER	SERV	CAL	FAT	CARB	FIB	PRO	

SNACK	SERV	CAL	FAT	CARB	FIB	PRO	

DAILY TOTALS		CAL	FAT	CARB	FIB	PRO	OTHER

EXERCISE	DURATION	INTENSITY	CALORIES BURNED

VITAMINS / QTY	SUPPLEMENTS / QTY	MEDICATIONS / QTY

DAILY JOURNAL

TODAY I FEEL:

DAY 25

DATE: DAY OF WEEK:

WATER INTAKE: ○   ○   ○   ○   ○   ○   ○   ○

BREAKFAST	SERV	CAL	FAT	CARB	FIB	PRO	OTHER

LUNCH	SERV	CAL	FAT	CARB	FIB	PRO	

DINNER	SERV	CAL	FAT	CARB	FIB	PRO	

SNACK	SERV	CAL	FAT	CARB	FIB	PRO	

DAILY TOTALS		CAL	FAT	CARB	FIB	PRO	OTHER

EXERCISE	DURATION	INTENSITY	CALORIES BURNED

VITAMINS / QTY	SUPPLEMENTS / QTY	MEDICATIONS / QTY

DAILY JOURNAL

TODAY I FEEL:

DAY 26

DATE:			DAY OF WEEK:				

WATER INTAKE: ○   ○   ○   ○   ○   ○   ○   ○

BREAKFAST	SERV	CAL	FAT	CARB	FIB	PRO	OTHER

LUNCH	SERV	CAL	FAT	CARB	FIB	PRO	

DINNER	SERV	CAL	FAT	CARB	FIB	PRO	

SNACK	SERV	CAL	FAT	CARB	FIB	PRO	

DAILY TOTALS		CAL	FAT	CARB	FIB	PRO	OTHER

EXERCISE	DURATION	INTENSITY	CALORIES BURNED

VITAMINS / QTY	SUPPLEMENTS / QTY	MEDICATIONS / QTY

DAILY JOURNAL

TODAY I FEEL:

DAY 27

DATE: DAY OF WEEK:

WATER INTAKE: ○   ○   ○   ○   ○   ○   ○   ○

BREAKFAST	SERV	CAL	FAT	CARB	FIB	PRO	OTHER

LUNCH	SERV	CAL	FAT	CARB	FIB	PRO	

DINNER	SERV	CAL	FAT	CARB	FIB	PRO	

SNACK	SERV	CAL	FAT	CARB	FIB	PRO	

DAILY TOTALS		CAL	FAT	CARB	FIB	PRO	OTHER

EXERCISE	DURATION	INTENSITY	CALORIES BURNED

VITAMINS / QTY	SUPPLEMENTS / QTY	MEDICATIONS / QTY

DAILY JOURNAL

TODAY I FEEL:

DAY 28

DATE: DAY OF WEEK:

WATER INTAKE: ○ ○ ○ ○ ○ ○ ○ ○

BREAKFAST	SERV	CAL	FAT	CARB	FIB	PRO	OTHER

LUNCH	SERV	CAL	FAT	CARB	FIB	PRO	

DINNER	SERV	CAL	FAT	CARB	FIB	PRO	

SNACK	SERV	CAL	FAT	CARB	FIB	PRO	

DAILY TOTALS		CAL	FAT	CARB	FIB	PRO	OTHER

EXERCISE	DURATION	INTENSITY	CALORIES BURNED

VITAMINS / QTY	SUPPLEMENTS / QTY	MEDICATIONS / QTY

DAILY JOURNAL

TODAY I FEEL:

DAY 29

DATE: DAY OF WEEK:

WATER INTAKE: ○   ○   ○   ○   ○   ○   ○   ○

BREAKFAST	SERV	CAL	FAT	CARB	FIB	PRO	OTHER

LUNCH	SERV	CAL	FAT	CARB	FIB	PRO	

DINNER	SERV	CAL	FAT	CARB	FIB	PRO	

SNACK	SERV	CAL	FAT	CARB	FIB	PRO	

DAILY TOTALS		CAL	FAT	CARB	FIB	PRO	OTHER

EXERCISE	DURATION	INTENSITY	CALORIES BURNED

VITAMINS / QTY	SUPPLEMENTS / QTY	MEDICATIONS / QTY

DAILY JOURNAL

TODAY I FEEL:

DAY 30

DATE:			DAY OF WEEK:				

WATER INTAKE: ○   ○   ○   ○   ○   ○   ○   ○

BREAKFAST	SERV	CAL	FAT	CARB	FIB	PRO	OTHER

LUNCH	SERV	CAL	FAT	CARB	FIB	PRO	

DINNER	SERV	CAL	FAT	CARB	FIB	PRO	

SNACK	SERV	CAL	FAT	CARB	FIB	PRO	

DAILY TOTALS		CAL	FAT	CARB	FIB	PRO	OTHER

EXERCISE	DURATION	INTENSITY	CALORIES BURNED

VITAMINS / QTY	SUPPLEMENTS / QTY	MEDICATIONS / QTY

DAILY JOURNAL

TODAY I FEEL:

Resources

GENERAL

Websites

American Heart Association, www.americanheart.org
nutrition.gov
usda.gov
mypyramid.gov
Harvard School of Public Health, www.hsph.harvard.edu

Books

Herbert, Victor, and Genell J. Subak-Sharpe, eds. *Total Nutrition: The Only Guide You'll Ever Need–From the Mount Sinai School of Medicine*. New York: St. Martin's Press, 1995.

Roizen, Michael F., M.D., and Mehmet C. Oz, M.D. *YOU: The Owner's Manual: An Insider's Guide to the Body That Will Make You Healthier and Younger*. New York: HarperCollins, 2005.

HIGH-FIBER FOODS

http://www.hsph.harvard.edu/nutritionsource/fiber.html
http://www.mayoclinic.com/health/high-fiber-foods/NU00582

NUTRITION INFORMATION

http://www.hsph.harvard.edu/nutritionsource/index.html
calorie-count.com

dietfacts.com
nutritiondata.com
calorieking.com

VEGETARIANS

Messina, Virginia, and Mark Messina. *The Vegetarian Way: Total Health
   for You and Your Family.* New York: Three Rivers Press, 1996.
Vesanto, Melina, and Brenda Davis. *The New Becoming Vegetarian: The
   Essential Guide to a Healthy Vegetarian Diet.* Summertown, Tenn.:
   Healthy Living Publications, 2003.

RESISTANCE EXERCISES

http://www.bodybuilding.com/fun/exercises.htm

Acknowledgments

I always thought that the term *self-made* was a strange way to describe anyone who had created success in his or her life, because there are very few people who actually accomplish anything significant without tremendous help from others. I am no exception.

My wife, Nikki, is the person who makes my life complete and keeps me balanced. Without her I would be a runaway train at times. I don't know why I was lucky enough to find her, but thank God I did.

Logan, unfortunately you are too young to read this, but when you finally can, I want you to know that you have been an unbelievable inspiration to me. Until you came along I had a very hard time realizing that anything was more important than me. Thanks for opening my eyes.

Thanks to my outstanding family—Dad, Mom, Tracy, Tina, Jamie, Jeremy, and Julie—for their input into this program and this book. For almost my entire life we really were the kings and queens of Fatland. We never had a lot of money or anything to brag about, but I always felt loved. If anyone can ever find a way to put what we have in a book, it could solve all of the world's problems. You are all fantastic.

Harry, I told you one day I would say thanks in a big way. I'm sure you thought I would send you a Ferrari or something. Who knows, though; maybe someday. Until then, thanks for being there when I needed family the most. It made all the difference.

I want to thank Elicia Hammond, Rachel Pierce, Pat & JT, and *Good Morning America* for helping me to get this story out. Special thanks to Kathy Sarantos-Niver for leading me to the next step that allowed us to turn our ideas into this book.

Thanks to John Burley for teaching me the concept of abundance and Keith Cunningham for teaching me about possibility.

Thanks to Elsa Dixon for her suggestions in the early stages of creation and thanks to Shaye Areheart and Julia Pastore for getting this project to the finish line.

Finally, I want to say thanks to my agent, Candice Fuhrman, for returning my call Friday before a long weekend. I will never forget your saying, "Finally, something new." You are a person who makes things happen and creates opportunities. Thank you so much.

Index

ABOUT THE AUTHOR

Tony Dean and his family live in Omaha, Nebraska. After the Dean family of eight had lost 500 pounds, they decided to make an impact on their community and helped a group from their home city lose 3,500 pounds. Now the Dean family is taking this crusade from city to city, helping people lose weight using the F.A.S.T. diet. Visit their website, **www.thefastdiet.net,** to find out how you can get involved—and become the next F.A.S.T. diet success story!